OUR STROKE of LUCK

OUR STROKE *of* LUCK

*New Technology
Enables Stroke Victims
to Make a Full*
RECOVERY

J. Gerry Purdy, PhD

New York

OUR STROKE *of* LUCK
New Technology Enables Stroke Victims to Make a Full RECOVERY

Published in New York, New York, by Morgan James Publishing. Morgan James and The Entrepreneurial Publisher are trademarks of Morgan James, LLC.
www.MorganJamesPublishing.com

The Morgan James Speakers Group can bring authors to your live event. For more information or to book an event visit The Morgan James Speakers Group at www.TheMorganJamesSpeakersGroup.com.

ISBN 978-1-68350-014-8 paperback
ISBN 978-1-68350-015-5 eBook
ISBN 978-1-68350-016-2 hardcover
Library of Congress Control Number:
2016905060

Cover Design by:
Rachel Lopez
www.r2cdesign.com

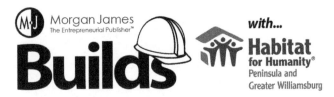

In an effort to support local communities, raise awareness and funds, Morgan James Publishing donates a percentage of all book sales for the life of each book to Habitat for Humanity Peninsula and Greater Williamsburg.

Get involved today! Visit
www.MorganJamesBuilds.com

DEDICATION

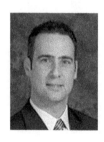

Raul G. Nogueira, M.D.
Director, Neuroendovascular Division
Marcus Stroke & Neuroscience Center
Grady Memorial Hospital, Atlanta, GA
Professor, Emory School of Medicine
Decatur, GA

This book is dedicated to Dr. Raul Nogueira. It was through his skill and experience and the 'luck of the draw" that he was allowed to use a new clot removal instrument to use a catheter to go into Alicia's right medial carotid artery (MCA) to extract most of the stroke-causing clot and, thus, return blood flow into the right side of Alicia's brain.

It's clear that Dr. Nogueira saved Alicia's life. Without him being available, Alicia most certainly would not be living a full, vibrant life now years after she suffered the stroke.

Dr. Nogueira was Principal Investigator for the stent retriever instrument that was approved by the FDA on August 15, 2012. Eventually, this instrument (and others like it) will be used by neurosurgeons all over the world to increase their success in removing stroke-causing clots and give ischemic stroke victims a chance to return to a fully functional life.

Naturally, the long term solution is through prevention but that will likely take a long time to achieve. About eighty percent of strokes are called '"ischemic" because they lodge in the brain and block blood from flowing. A smaller twenty percent of strokes are due to rupture of arteries in the brain. While blood clots can be "bad" when they travel freely usually from the heart into the brain, most blood clots are "good" because they enable us to heal quickly from any cut or surgical wound.

If we prevented clots from forming, there would be a bigger danger of bleeding to death from a simple cut. In a dream world, we'd like to keep the "good" clots and eliminate the "bad" clots which might not be possible. However, it might be possible to reduce or prevent "bad" clots from owing to conditions such as atrial fibrillation.

We commend the work being done by Dr. Raul Nogueira and look forward to continuing to use their innovative procedures to help bring loved ones afflicted with ischemic strokes back to life while researchers work on the longer term problem of preventing them from happening in the first place.

TABLE OF CONTENTS

	Foreword	*ix*
	Acknowledgements	*xv*
	Preface	*xxvii*

Chapter 1	Innocence	1
Chapter 2	Quick: Define a Stroke	6
Chapter 3	Calm before the Storm	11
Chapter 4	Stroke Day: August 23, 2011	20
Chapter 5	Grady Stroke Center	38
Chapter 6	"Why did this happen to me?"	59
Chapter 7	Returning Home	69
Chapter 8	Becoming Overwhelmed	83
Chapter 9	Rehabilitation	95
Chapter 10	Back in the Saddle Again	103
Chapter 11	Trying to Figure Out What Happened	128
Chapter 12	A Healthy but Slightly Different Person	136
Chapter 13	Our Stroke of Luck	152
Chapter 14	Personal Reflections	164
Chapter 15	Bibliography	170

FOREWORD

by
Michael Frankel, MD
Director, Marcus Stroke Center
Grady Hospital
Atlanta, Georgia

Alicia Purdy was going to be another victim. When I met her she was completely paralyzed on her left side, unaware that she was weak and unaware that she was having a stroke that could kill her. For 25 years I have watched the extreme personal devastation of stroke. But Alicia's inspirational story of triumph gives us a light in the tunnel, a glimpse of what is truly possible when people come together to help each other in a community. It is a great honor for me to set the stage for her story which played out in a public hospital setting, a place where few people consider cutting edge treatment to be possible.

As a young resident in the field of neurology, I witnessed patients of all ages become victim to the tragedy of life altering disability and death from stroke, often times affecting people in the prime of their lives, people with families who need them, people like Alicia. Far too often, I could offer nothing more than a comforting hand and stand by as the hand of fate determined whether a patient would recover. Such helpless feelings for a young physician were disturbing. Although I had years of education and training in the specialized field of neurology. I had no way to alter the course of the most common cause of serious long-term adult disability.

As I emerged from training and considered a faculty position at Emory University, I found myself with a choice. There were no proven treatments for stroke. The research in animals could not be replicated in humans. Doctors of neurology were labeled as those who would "diagnose and adios." However, new hope was emerging from the labs of Justin Zivin, an internationally renowned neuroscientist with new ideas and proof that a drug used for heart attack victims, tissue plasminogen activator (tPA), could help people with stroke.

But neurologists are notorious for being nihilistic, thinking that few or no treatments exist for a disease. This belief is largely borne from diseases like stroke that had no proven treatment despite years of extensive research. Like a search for the needle in the haystack, a solution was elusive.

When I started my career at Emory, I became aware of a new study of tPA in patients with stroke. Built on the seminal work of Dr. Zivin and others, a large clinical trial was being put together. I was asked whether I wanted to be the Principal Investigator at Emory for the eight center studies across the US. At the time, I was inexperienced in research and had no idea what level of commitment it would take. My colleagues in neurology were nihilistic about the project because of published data referencing terrible outcomes from using similar clot-busting drugs like streptokinase in patients with stroke, and because of their personal experience with tPA when given for a heart attack.

Neurologists do not treat patients with heart attacks and are called to see the patient only if there is a neurologic problem. Even though tPA for heart attack causes bleeding into the brain less than one percent of the time, the neurologist gets called to see the patient only when this terrible complication occurs. Thus, the neurologist's perspective on tPA was that it was a terrible drug to be used for patients with stroke since it caused so much cerebral hemorrhage.

I would describe it as extreme cynicism amongst neurologists. A study of tPA in stroke was considered radical and dangerous. Yet, the data from Dr. Zivin was compelling. And two small-dose finding studies in people were encouraging. In my view, it was time to do the larger study.

We created the first 24/7 acute stroke team in the southeastern U.S. to meet the needs of this new study. The "team" was a study nurse and me, along with a great group of young neurology residents in training. I was on-call 24/7 for over two years, identifying potential candidates for treatment, obtaining written consent, and enrolling them into the study called the "NINDS tPA Stroke Trial." I did not know where it would lead, but I was very proud to be a part of such an important project, working alongside icons in the field like Thomas Brott at the University of Cincinnati and James Grotta at the University of Texas in Houston.

But my wife Kathi was just as unaware as I was of the commitment it would take to make this study work in Atlanta. There were many nights when, after my being up several nights in a row, Kathi would answer the phone for me in the middle of the night and screen the patient for possible enrollment with the physician seeing the patient in Grady's emergency room.

There were eight academic centers participating in the study which included forty-one hospitals across the US. Our center primarily utilized Grady Hospital which was the fifth leading recruiting site in the country, a feat that no one thought possible since Grady is a safety-net hospital with limited resources and is not felt to have the capability of cutting edge research and care that a major academic center hospital can provide. But we showed that it could be done.

For our team, the feeling of offering a possible cure for stroke was exhilarating. But because the study was double blind (we didn't know whether the patient was getting tPA or a placebo solution of saline), there was no way to tell whether the drug was working. Many patients were improving, but we didn't know whether it was the drug or not. And we weren't allowed to find out until the three year study was concluded.

On a day I'll never forget in August of 1995, the eight principal investigators from across the U.S gathered in Virginia to review the data from the study of 624 patients at the end of the project. The project officer at the NIH, Dr. John Marler, had just seen the data a few days earlier. His first slide was a picture of four aces. It was his way of saying that tPA was highly effective on all four measures of success as defined at the start of the study.

But the nihilist and naysayers remained skeptical about the results, even though they were published in the most prestigious journal, the New England Journal of Medicine. Some thought the eight principal investigators were paid by the drug company Genentech, the maker of tPA, during the study to alter the results in some nefarious way. As we gathered in Bethesda for the press conference to announce the findings in December of 1995, the week the New England Journal of Medicine paper was to be published, we found ourselves in front of a large room of reporters ready to ask questions. "How many of you have stock in Genentech?" one reporter from ABC news asked. "None of us" was the reply. Another asked, "What will this mean for patients with stroke?" We were not sure at the time, but we were sure it was going to be a revolution in how the disease would be treated from that moment forward.

In June of 1996, the FDA approved tPA to be used in patients with stroke who present within three hours of symptom onset. But despite the approval, few physicians were willing to use it. So we began working with hospitals in Georgia to help them understand the data and S them in building their own stroke teams. These were launched in 2000 when we designed the Georgia Coverdell Stroke Registry, a project funded by the Centers for Disease Control and Prevention (CDC) to assist hospitals in collecting data and using it to improve stroke care. We amassed a group of forty randomly selected hospitals and began a project that continues to this day, now with over sixty participating.

But as Alicia lay unaware of her paralyzed left side, not moving her left arm or leg, and looking calm in the midst of disaster (a terrible trick the brain plays on us when the right side of the brain is injured by stroke), I thought about how far we had come from the days of tPA.

The day that Alicia appeared at the Marcus Stroke & Neuroscience Center, we were in the early stages of forging a new era in stroke care. The new drug tPA was now being used as a standard of care throughout Georgia and the U.S. Our work had translated into saving countless lives. But because of the narrow window of treatment, few people were eligible since most did not arrive to the hospital in time.

New data was emerging about specialized catheters that were small and flexible enough to remove the blood clots blocking the arteries in the brain during an acute stroke. Watching the field of vascular neurology evolve as cardiology did 20 years prior, I could see that we were on the verge of radically changing the field of treatment, much like we did with tPA years earlier.

I was fortunate to pitch my idea to a new CEO, Mike Young, in 2009. In his first week of taking on one of the most challenging hospital leadership positions in the U.S., Mike was set in motion to lead Grady from near financial collapse into a new era of success and sustainability. My idea was to build the greatest stroke center in the world. At the time, no one believed it could be done, particularly at a public hospital like Grady. But Mike listened and agreed – it was time.

My career has been punctuated by people telling me what was impossible and then finding a way to make it possible. That was certainly true of tPA. And, it was also true of the center we were about to build – the Marcus Stroke & Neuroscience Center.

Through the generous gift of Bernie Marcus, a Home Depot co-founder, we constructed a world class state-of-the-art facility for patients with stroke. We built the world's first neurocritical intensive care unit (ICU) that contains an angiogram suite, a place where inside-out (called endovascular) surgery on brain arteries is performed. Placing the operating room for endovascular surgery in the ICU was considered radical. And yes, it was also considered impossible.

We then set in motion a plan to attract the very best physicians in the U.S. to join us. A world class facility, the support of a dynamic CEO and leadership at Emory University were all key factors in building an A-team that would bring cutting edge therapeutics to the bedside on every patient and serve as Atlanta's regional destination site for patients with acute stroke.

Upon arrival, Alicia was seen by our team and immediately taken to the endovascular suite. The rest of her story is best told by her and her husband, Gerry Purdy. It is an amazing story of triumph and love.

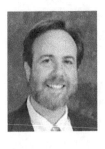

Michael Frankel, M.D.
Director, Marcus Stroke Center
Grady Hospital
Atlanta, Georgia
Professor of Director of Vascular Neurology
Emory Medical School
Decatur, Georgia

ACKNOWLEDGEMENTS

I could not have written this book without a lot of assistance from a number of people. Most important, of course, are the people in the medical profession who helped treat Alicia's stroke. Without their assistance, Alicia would not have been able to make a full recovery. Some additional people also assisted in Alicia's rehabilitation. I need to also acknowledge members of our families, Alicia's personal and equestrian friends and supporters, and the people who took the time to edit the book and make me look better than I am as a writer.

Medical Support

There are a number of people in the medical community that were directly or indirectly involved with helping Alicia recover from her stroke. These include: Raul Nogueira, M.D., Emory Medical School and Marcus Stroke Center, Michael Frankel, M.D., Emory Medical School and Marcus Stroke Center, Lisa Rivera, M.D., Neurologist Resident, Marcus Stroke Center, Randolph P. Martin, M.D., Cardiologist,

Piedmont Heart Institute, Atlanta and family friend, David Dubose, M.D., concierge physician and family friend, Matt Burrell, M.D., GYN oncology physician and family friend, Northside Hospital Emergency Room Staff (who administered tPA), Paul Harris, M.D., attending physician in the Northside Emergency Room, Gerald Silverboard, M.D., attending Neurologist (who referred Alicia to Grady Stroke Center), Meredith Bell, M.D., attending Radiologist (who spotted the clot in the MCA artery via MRI images), Serge Ouanounou, M.D., Radiologist who also read the MRI and reported the results to Dr. Silverboard and Bernie Marcus who provided financial support to create the Marcus Stroke Center at Grady Hospital.

Rehabilitation
We had additional support during rehabilitation including: Northside Hospital Rehabilitation Department, Linda Kumar, Core Pilates, Genna Brown (helped Alicia around the house and ran errands).

Family
I want to thank the members of Alicia's family including Bruce and Carol Grant, daughter Sandy and son-in-law Grant as well as her son Grant. Likewise, members of my family helped Alicia in her recovery. These included Jill and Paul Sarkozi, Kristi Riggs, Bryan and Claudia Purdy, Jason and Emma Purdy as well as Jennifer and Doug Meads.

Equestrian Community
There were many people in the equestrian community that supported Alicia both before and after her stroke. These include: Cathy Whiteside, horse trainer (with Greta), Julie Curtin, horse trainer, and all the riders and support staff at New Vintage Farm, Woodstock, Georgia (with Polina), Amy Barrett, Assistant Trainer, New Vintage Farm, Karen and Dal Franchen, New Vintage Farm, John Roper, trainer (with Polina),

Kelly Mullen, rider & trainer (with Polina), Jerry and Barbara Goldsmith (owned Greta), Susan Tuccinardi, Castlewood Farm, Wellington (with Ella), Carol Dollard, Steeplechase Farm, Wellington (with Polina), Anne Cheatham, Sarah Ingram, Theresa and Albert Meneffee, Amy Smith, Liz Sponseller and Bonnie and Chico Zarate.

Friends

We are very fortunate to have many friends who gave support for Alicia in her recovery. These included: Connie and Frank Blythe, Tina Brown, Nancy Bulls, Janet Burrell, Sherri and Jess Crawford, Mynnel Yates DuBois, Eleanor and Bill Effinger, Lynn and Allan Ford, Kathy Foster & Mike Nelson, Wendy and Bob Gifford, Danielle Goldberg, Trena and Robert Hargraves, Linda Keefe, Peggy and Bill Knight, Nina and Keith MacRae, Tom and Sharron Marshall, Mary Portman and Jim Adams, Kathy and Jerry Sands, Lynn and Bill Schroeder, Tamara Stewart, Susan and Chip Traynor, Cecilia and Allan Wright and John and Maggie Vespico.

Publishing

I am indebted to the following people who helped with editing and publishing the book. These include: Vivian Booth, copy editing, Lindy Rogers, copy editing, Jill Sarkozi, copy editing and story line recommendations and David Handcock & Megan Malone, Morgan James Publishing.

Song Lyrics

Preface, Page xxvi

"I ain't here for a long time
I'm here for a good time"

Song: "Here for a Good Time"

Chapter 3, Page 11
"I will wait, I will wait for you."

Chapter 3, Page 11 (second lyric quote)
"Haven't seen you since high school
Good to see you're still beautiful"

Chapter 4, Page 20
"I would love to fix it all for you … We all got bruises."

Song: "Bruises"
Group: Train featuring Ashley Monroe
Album: California 37 (2012)
Words and Music by Pat Monahan, Espen Lind and Amund Bjorklund

Chapter 5, Page 38
"I had a dream so big and loud
I jumped so high I touched the clouds.
Wo-o-o-o-oh [2x]
I stretched my hands out to the sky
We danced with monsters through the night
Wo-o-o-o-oh [2x]
This is going to be the best day of my life."

Song: "Best Day of My Life"

Chapter 6, Page 59
"Just give me a reason
Just a little bit's enough"

Song: "Just Give Me a Reason"
Group: PINK with fun.'s lead singer Nate Ruess
Album: The Truth About Love ((2013)
Words and Music by Alecia Moore, Jeff Bhasker and Nate Ruess

Chapter 7, Page 69
"And all along I believed I would find you
Time has brought your heart to me
I have loved you for a thousand years
I'll love you for a thousand more"

Song: "A Thousand Years"
Group: Christina Perri & David Hodges (2011)
Album: The Twilight Saga: Breaking Dawn – Part 1
Words and Music by David Hodges and Christina Perri
Copyright (c) 2011 EMI Blackwood Music Inc., 12:06 Publishing, Miss
Perri Lane Publishing and Warner-Tamerlane Publishing Corp.
All Rights on behalf of EMI Blackwood Music Inc. and 12:06 Publishing
Administered by Sony/ATV Music Publishing LLC, 424 Church Street,
Suite 1200, Nashville, TN 37219
All Rights on behalf of Miss Perri Lane Publishing Controlled and
Administered by Songs Of Kobalt Music Publishing
International Copyright Secured All Rights Reserved
Reprinted by Permission of Hal Leonard LLC and Alfred Music

Chapter 8, Page 83
"I'm only a man in a silly red sheet
Digging for kryptonite on this one way street
Only a man in a funny red sheet
Looking for special things inside of me
Inside of me, inside of me."

Song: "Superman (It's Not Easy)"
Group: Five for Fighting
Album: America Town
Words and Music by John Ondrasik

Chapter 9, Page 95
"Missed the Saturday dance
Heard they crowded the floor
Couldn't bear it without you
Don't get around much anymore"

Chapter 10, Page 103
"Whoopi-ty-aye-oh
Rockin' to and fro
Back in the saddle again
Whoopi-ty-aye-yay
I go my way
Back in the saddle again"

Song: "Back in the Saddle Again"
Group: Gene Autry & Ray Whitley
Album: Gene Autry's Western Classics album (1947)
Also used in the 1993 movie, "Sleepless in Seattle" Soundtrack
Words and Music by Gene Autry and Ray Whitley
© 1939 (Renewed) Gene Autry's Western Music Publishing Co. and
Katielu Music
All Rights Reserved Used by Permission
Reprinted by Permission of Hal Leonard LLC

Chapter 11, Page 128
"I wanna thank you very much
Thank you for lending me love
Now I'm levitating
Cos I feel like I've been waiting
For a lifetime
For your touch"

Song: "Thank you"
Group: Westlife
Album: Turnaround (November 2003)
Words and Music by Simon Perry, Steve Mac and Wayne Hector

[Note: This was the music used for the First Dance at our wedding, October 4, 2008]

Chapter 12, Page 136
"Days like these lead to...
Nights like this lead to
Love like ours.
You light the spark in my bonfire heart."

Song: "Bonfire Heart"
Group: James Blunt
Album: Moon Landing (2013)
Words and Music by James Blunt and Ryan Teflder

Chapter 13, Page 153
"Some guys have all the luck
Some guys have all the pain
Some guys get all the breaks"

Song: "Some Guys Have All The Luck"
Group: Rod Stewart
Album: Camouflage (1984)
Arrangement by Rod Stewart
Words and Music by Jeff Fortgang

PREFACE

"I ain't here for a long time
I'm here for a good time"

George Strait, *Here for a Good Time*
Reprinted by Permission.

I wrote this book for two reasons. First, I wanted to help other caregivers who have had a loved one or a close friend afflicted by a stroke. Second, I wanted to tell a great story of hope – the story of my wife Alicia Purdy's stroke and recovery. I wanted to let people know that it is possible with good timing, skilled neurosurgery and rehabilitation to get the person you love back to a fully recovered or "normal" state.

Many of you likely think that I am kidding, rationalizing or trivializing a terrible situation because most of the time when people run into someone who has had a stroke, it is very noticeable. The stroke victims are either are partially paralyzed or cannot talk normally (or both). I often call this the Frankenstein effect since their condition is so noticeable.

Alicia's brain was compromised by the clot that formed the stroke, but because it was removed relatively quickly after the clot traveled to her brain, she was able to return to a normal, productive life. People need to know that such a recovery is possible, and, over the coming years, we're going to see more people like Alicia beat debilitating effects of a stroke.

While not everyone who has a stroke will have the same outcome as Alicia, she serves as a shining example (or "Poster Child") for others that full recovery is possible. We hope that what may be an unusual, amazing case today will become an everyday occurrence in the future.

There are a number of books that have been written by stroke victims. Kirk Douglas wrote a book called <u>My Stroke of Luck</u> about his stroke and recovery. A friend of mine, Jeff Kagan, wrote <u>Life After Stroke</u> that gives a wonderful account of his thoughts and feelings during his multi-year recovery from an ischemic stroke that afflicted the left side of his brain (Alicia's stroke was on the right side of her brain). Dr. Jill Bolte Taylor wrote an account of her stroke in a <u>My Stroke of Insight</u>. And, there's <u>The Fat Lady Sang</u> by Robert Evans, famous movie actor and producer, who suffered a series of three successive strokes in 1998. You can find all of these books online in either paper or digital forms.

I encourage everyone to learn more about strokes and, in particular, the early warning signs. Strokes can be managed successfully if you take action quickly. It is far better to go to the emergency room worrying that you or your loved one is experiencing a stroke than it is to wait and react once the damage has been done. Literally, just an hour or two can make a huge difference in the outcome.

If a friend or loved one experiences a stroke, you will have to deal with a number of issues once they are released from the hospital. Many people are now being treated early enough that they will, over time, return to being almost the same as before they had their stroke. Truly, they are "normal" by every measure, but are not exactly the same normal as before. I describe this in more detail in the following chapters.

Be sure to share this book with your friends and family. If someone you know or a loved one happens to begin having a stroke, you will be better able to recognize the symptoms and seek skilled medical attention quickly. Being able to recognize early the symptoms of a stroke will definitely reduce or eliminate serious long-term effects.

And remember, you are <u>not</u> likely to say, "Hey guys, I think I'm having a stroke." That's because your brain simply can't recognize the symptoms. If you're having a stroke, your mind does not feel any pain. You might not be able to move correctly or at all, but your mind will not think of it as a stroke. It takes the people around you to recognize that something is wrong and to seek medical attention as soon as possible.

My hope is that you will give this book to those you love. They will learn how to recognize early the onset of a stroke and by getting the person afflicted to a stroke center quickly. That one small thing will undoubtedly extend that person's life by many years.

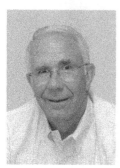

Know how to recognize the onset of a stroke. It may save the life of someone you know or love.

J. Gerry Purdy, Ph.D.
Wellington, Florida
gerry.purdy@gmail.com

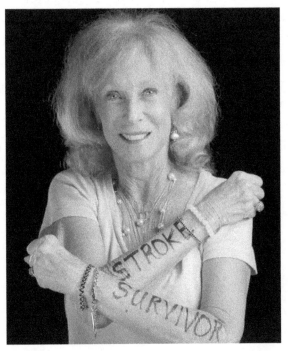

Credit: Robert X. Fogarty, Dear World, with permission. Photo taken on October 22, 2014 at the UNIFY analyst meeting in Scottsdale, Arizona.

Chapter 1

INNOCENCE

Where were you the morning of Sept. 11, 2001? Anyone old enough to remember can tell you the exact instant that they heard about the attack on the World Trade Center in New York City. One second, you are living your normal (rather innocent) life, and the next second, everything changes.

That is the way it is with strokes. One minute you are going through life just as you have for years without a worry in the world (other than the normal everyday things like dealing with you kids, career and money) and a few minutes later your world changes drastically.

But, instead of the obvious trauma from an auto accident or a heart attack, this one silently creeps up on you without any warning signs. Even when you experience the onset of a stroke, you are not aware that anything is wrong. This is not a situation in which you yell out, "Oh no! I'm having a stroke! Help!" Rather, you have no idea anything is wrong and then someone you know might say to you, "What's wrong with you? I think something is wrong. Let's go to the emergency room to let them check on you."

Or, the situation might be reversed: you observe someone who seems a bit off. They might be slurring words when they have not been drinking or they might appear confused. Or, they might say they have suddenly become dizzy. You might ask them if they are OK, but because the person suffering a stroke does not have the capacity to judge that a stroke is in process, it might require your intervention and getting that person to an emergency room so a medical assessment can be made.

The signs of a stroke are a little ambiguous. It is not that there are not real signs, but, rather, they are not definitive and they do not indicate just how serious the problem is. They could be the signs of something else, but you are always better off taking action even if you think, "What's all the fuss? I've just had one glass of wine. I feel a little light-headed and will go sit down for a few minutes. It's nothing. Don't be so concerned!" It costs far less to go to the emergency room thinking that the person you care about may be having a stroke when, in fact, it may be something else. If you do not take action when they are, indeed, having a stroke, then the cost to both the victim's life and to the family financially could be huge.

Now, let's take a look at the Stroke Association warning signs for a stroke:

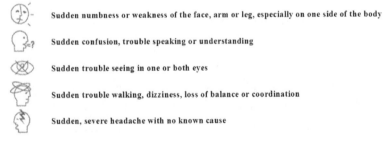

Figure 1-1. Signs of a Stroke

If you look at any one of these things, you might think, "Why, I have short-term memory loss all the time. We all have to live with it."

Or, it is not uncommon to have a headache out of the blue. Or, you might feel that your eyes are a little blurry or feel a little dizzy or lose your balance. You might not think anything of it, but family and friends around you will certainly notice that "Something isn't right." Listen to them. Do not reject what they are saying.

Or, perhaps you notice something is not right with one of your friends. You should not hold back. Rather, you should confront the friend and let them know you are concerned. You may have to take them to the emergency room to see if something is more serious such as a stroke.

Of course, if there are multiple warning signs at the same time, then you need to get help as quickly as possible. Again, it may be that you are the one who notices multiple warning signs in someone else. Then, you should not hesitate. You should get them to an emergency room as soon as possible.

Another thing about strokes: while there are some conditions that pre-dispose people to having a stroke, it is possible to have a stroke without any pre-disposition. I know this for a fact as my wife Alicia is the epitome of health for someone her age. She is thin, exercises regularly, has low cholesterol (and very high HDL), does not smoke and watches her diet. Alicia is likely the last person in the world that you would think would have a stroke. But, in fact, she did and it came on without any warning.

Also, while strokes are more prevalent in older people, young people have strokes, too. Thus, it's possible for anyone at any age to suffer a stroke. I call it the "silent affliction" because it comes on without warning, is not painful and, yet, can result in debilitating lifelong paralysis.

I truly wish there was a way that everyone could be "less innocent" about strokes and have the same awareness that society has regarding heart attacks. I hope, this book will provide one small step in that direction.

If we are all a little less innocent, then we will be more likely to get people assistance and treatment before it is too late. Over-reaction is far better than avoidance or delay. Sure, there are times that people are alone for long periods that make it difficult to recognize the onset of a stroke, like when a spouse is out of town or away from home that may delay the detection of the onset of a stroke. There are a number of companies that are providing sensors with remote access to we can monitor our loved ones and make sure they are all right.

However, most of the time, we are around other people during the day and night. It is at these times when the signs of stroke hit without warning that we can recognize what is happening and react quickly.

You will likely have someone you know suffer a stroke. While the realization that it is a serious situation can be alarming and disconcerting, it is far better to feel scared and do something than it is not to recognize the seriousness of the situation and do nothing or believe that nothing is wrong.

Do not be innocent. Be aware. If a stroke happens, there are resources that can minimize the effects, but if you do not act quickly, you could put yourself or the person afflicted at risk of having more serious long-term effects.

I was innocent about strokes but fortunately, I was able to quickly get help in time for my wife Alicia. I was scared out of my mind, but once I realized what was happening, I wanted to utilize every possible resource in the world to help her recover and live a productive life.

Here is a good mental image to think about if you realize that someone is having a stroke: think of a clock that starts counting down from 10 hours to zero. You are in a race to beat the clock. If you get help initial help within hours, you can expect to have a good chance at a positive outcome (providing it is a clot-based stroke that can benefit from available treatment). It is the Olympic gun going off and it is your job to "dash like hell" to seek help and assistance.

NOTE TO READERS

The rest of this book contains some very emotionally intense experiences. It will elicit strong emotions in you. You may cry and may even laugh at times. This book allows you to peek into someone's life who experienced a stroke and to experience for yourself what it is like to deal with the situation.

My wife, Alicia, suffered a stroke on Tuesday evening, August 23, 2011. It was a life threatening situation. And yet, we had a wonderful, positive outcome because we were lucky enough to have responded quickly and to have some of the best resources in the world available to us that facilitated a positive outcome.

Chapter 2

QUICK: DEFINE A STROKE

Heart attack!

Quick – think about what your mind conjures up when you see these two words. You know what a heart attack is. You know it's often lethal. You know it's painful. If anyone around you has a heart attack, you're immediately aware of it.

You think, "Oh my God, he (or she) is having a heart attack! Call 911! Administer CPR!" You might not have had training to administer CPR, but you may have seen it done on TV. Here are the basics: You make sure their airway is open in their mouth, you breath into their mouth covering their nose with your fingers (so the air will go into their lungs and not back out their nose) and then push on the person's sternum. It is often referred to as "ABC": create or open the Airway, Breath into their mouth to force air into their lungs and push on their Chest to help with circulation.

Because of all the publicity about heart attacks, most of the public know what to do when someone has a heart attack. And, even if they are unsure, they can at least recognize what is happening so they can solicit help from people nearby. You may get nervous yourself just standing there, even if you are not directly administering CPR. But, you know the general idea of what to do. You know the person needs help very quickly or he/she will likely die.

I remember when I was walking around Chastain Park in Atlanta with my Dachshund, Fritzie, in 2008 when I came around a corner to find a few people helping a jogger who had clearly had a heart attack. He was lying on the sidewalk and others were giving CPR. Someone had called 911 and I could hear sirens in the distance. The person regained consciousness, but was told to stay still. He related that he had pains in his left arm.

The emergency response team was there in less than four minutes and immediately checked his heart on a portable heart monitor. They inserted a catheter in his arm. They took his blood pressure. They confirmed with medical support that it was likely a heart attack, and they quickly got him onto a stretcher and into the ambulance.

I remember standing there not really able to do anything directly for the jogger who was lying on the sidewalk although I did help manage some of the traffic congestion that had stopped to "rubber neck" to see what had happened. I can remember my heart pounding and feeling nervous. It was a scary situation. Fortunately, the collapsed runner looked to be stable.

About two weeks later, I was walking in the park again and saw someone who had also been present at the time of the runner collapsing. I asked if he knew what had happened to the jogger. He said he knew him and that he had triple by-pass surgery and was now doing great.

I mention these things about heart attacks because they serve as a good example of situations that happen in your life in which you may be uncomfortable and/or scared, but, at the same time, you have a general sense of what is happening and what to do about it. It is not like, "What the hell is going on here?" You know what is happening and generally what to do.

Now, let us take a very different kind of situation. You approach a man who is sitting on a bench. He looks relatively normal. He is staring straight ahead and appears to not be focusing on anything. He looks to be in a stupor. The person is not expressing any pain. He has not passed out. He is not yelling for help. Unless you knew the person, you would likely just pass him by and not think anything of it.

But these are some of the warning signs of someone having a stroke. Already, you can see that these indicators are very different from a heart attack, but the public does not typically have much education, awareness or sensitivity to someone having a stroke.

If someone yelled out, "Stroke!" – would you know what to do? Or, even more importantly, would you recognize someone who is having a stroke? More than likely, you would feel a sense of dissonance: you would see a person that does not appear to be in any pain or distress, but someone is yelling "Stroke!" You are not sure what that to do. It conjures up an image of someone who is paralyzed on one side of their body. You see that all the time, but this person does not look like person who is hobbling around. Rather, they are not really doing anything.

That is what makes strokes so different from heart attacks. The person who is having a stroke does not typically realize it because there is not any pain. The brain does not have pain receptors so if something goes wrong in the brain, there is no immediate sense that something is wrong. Thus, if the stroke victim is not showing signs of distress, no one runs to help, administers CPR or calls 911. No life-saving call-to-action was requested and, unfortunately, none is often taken.

What often happens is that someone who knows the stroke victim realizes that the victim is not "normal." Their speech has suddenly become slurred or that half of their face is not working or that they cannot get up. The feeling of urgency creeps up on you: there is not any crescendo event with yelling, screaming and pain. You sense something is wrong and then it begins to occur to you that the person may be suffering a stroke. It is at that point, that you begin to feel fear and seek medical help and assistance.

Most of us – including this author – have never experienced someone having a stroke. You do not easily recognize it, and when you finally do, you are even more uncertain what to do about it, including whether to do CPR or take other life-saving measures.

Sure, you recognize the symptoms later – the appearance of what I call "The Frankenstein effect" where the victim walks with a shuffled gate, one arm dangling and one side of their mouth tilted or, worse, open and drooping. These are the stroke victims who did not get assistance fast enough or, if they did, the clot was inaccessible with today's technology. But, what if you saw someone who looked to be normal and then were told that they had suffered a full, devastating stroke? You would not believe it was possible, but this book demonstrates that someone can return to normal following having a stroke. It might be a slightly different 'normal' but no one looking at or talking with that person would know. "You're kidding, right?" is the most typical response. You can recover from a stroke, but it requires a series of events that must happen within a few hours. You are never prepared for something like this to happen. And, you typically are not aware that it is happening when it does.

This book is about what happened to me when I discovered that my wife had something wrong with her. I was not trained to recognize the onset of a stroke or what to do if someone began suffering a stroke. I simply was not prepared. In the end, we were just lucky that the timing of my arriving back home, the relatively quick recognition by the medical staff and the subsequent treatment were lined up just right.

It often doesn't end up this way. But, if more people knew the signs, then more people would end up like my wife, Alicia.

There are over seven hundred thousand people who suffer a stroke each year. Most people likely think the number is far less because you do not see stroke victims very often out in public, but when you do, they are quite noticeable. You will likely think, "God, that's just terrible." And, if they did not get professional medical assistance in time, being permanently disabled is often the result.

As you will find out from reading this book, it is possible to make a full recovery from a stroke due to very recent improvements in technology that enable trained neurosurgeons to find the clot that caused the stroke and remove it. This recent development results in many people who suffer a stroke to make a full recovery – something that would not have seemed possible just a few years ago.

Strokes affect a large number of family and friends in addition to the more than seven hundred thousand stroke victims. It certainly is likely every stroke victim will directly affect more than ten other people. Thus, over seven million people are indirectly affected by strokes every year. Most of us will likely know someone who has suffered a stroke at some point in their life. Therefore, it is important to know more about strokes and be able to help family and friends achieve more positive outcomes by acting quickly when someone appears to be having a stroke.

My wife Alicia and I had a dream life. Nothing was wrong with Alicia medically. There were no signs of a pending life threatening situation. Before I go into what happened to Alicia when I realized she was having stroke, I want to tell you the story about us and how we got together. It is a story of magic, coincidence, premonitions and romance that few would ever experience in their lives.

Read about the calm before the storm.

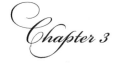

CALM BEFORE THE STORM

"I will wait, I will wait for you."

Mumford & Sons, *I Will Wait*
Reprinted by permission.

*"Haven't seen you since high school
Good to see you're still beautiful"*

Train featuring Ashley Monroe, *Bruises*
Reprinted by permission.

My wife, Alicia, and I dated for two years at Northside High School in Atlanta from 1959-1961. We were together most every day either at school or dating on the weekend. It was one of the first really serious relationships either of us had, and I thought we would likely be together for the rest of our lives.

After graduation, Alicia decided to go to the University of Georgia's Journalism School majoring in advertising and public relations. I started with a track scholarship at Clemson University but transferred over Christmas break in December 1962 to the University of Tennessee. Figure 1 shows Alicia and me at a dance at Northside High School in the fall of 1961. She is petite and gorgeous. I am one heck of a happy and lucky guy.

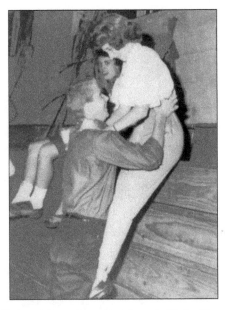

Figure 3-1 – Gerry Purdy and Alicia Grant
at a Northside High School dance, fall 1961.

When you begin to date as a teenager, you do not know if the person you are dating is a perfect match for you or not. You simply do not have the experience of dating enough to be certain. We both found out later that our relationship was clearly the best one we had in our lives. It took many years for us to realize that.

Alicia loved to ride horses, and her parents purchased a horse called Sky Parade for her to use during her junior and senior year at Northside High School in Atlanta. I would often go with her to see her ride in a horse show, either at Chastain Park or, occasionally, out of town at a nearby horse show in North or South Carolina. She tried to ride while at UGA but college life was too demanding.

We tried to see each other during our freshman year at college, but we slowly drifted apart. From my view, we did not have any cell phones, emails or texting. My rationalization is that if we had had these technologies, Alicia and I would have stayed in touch with each other and most likely would have gotten back together at some earlier time. Alicia felt we needed some time to grow up.

An amazing and strange sequence of events got us back together forty-five years later in 2006 – at a time in which both of us were in the process of getting a divorce. Each of us experienced premonitions about each other which then led to us communicating and getting back together in the summer of 2006.

My first premonition came in the March 2006 when I was diagnosed with sleep apnea. I did not realize it was a premonition at the time, but later I realized it was clearly connected to our getting back together. I had been suffering from sleep apnea for many years and went to have a sleep study done at Camino Medical Group in Cupertino in early 2006. The study showed that I was waking up an average of 30 times an hour during the night. There is a simple treatment for most people afflicted with sleep apnea: a Continuous Positive Augmented Pressure (CPAP) machine that simply adds air pressure to keep your nasal airwaves open while you sleep.

When I met with my sleep doctor, Alison Chen, she told me there would be two phases of improvement resulting from using a CPAP machine and, thus, being able to sleep all night: one would be immediate and the other delayed around one hundred days after I started using the CPAP at night. Sure enough, I found myself less sleepy during the day and more rested and almost like being shocked that I was not tired all day long as I had been for many, many years. I now sleep more at night and experience higher quality sleep getting in to Stage 2 and Stage 3 (deep) sleep, something that I hardly experienced before.

Because I had lacked the ability to experience deeper sleep, a lot of things started to readjust in my brain. Dr. Chen had told me that I would experience another major change about 100 days after I started to use my CPAP at night. This second change became my first premonition. She told me that about 100 days (plus or minus) after starting to use a CPAP at night, most people experience some life changes. The changes are not predictable or only in one area. Some people experience a small change such as a change in a habit. Others may experience a more significant change as in starting a new hobby and a few experience a significant change such as changing jobs or moving. She said that her research at Stanford and from other sleep studies seem to suggest that as the brain gets healthier, things that are important in your life come into focus.

I honestly did not pay any attention to her comment for a number of months because I had been so refreshed from finally sleeping all night. But, it was almost exactly 100 days later that Alicia and I started communicating with each other. Total coincidence? I think there was something going on in my brain's readjustment that resulted in my reaching out to my high school sweetheart. I am very thankful to Dr. Chen for her diagnosis and prescribing a CPAP to treat my sleep apnea. It is partly due to her that Alicia and I are now back together.

There was another stranger and a more outright premonition. I had been reading Audrey Niffenegger's Time Traveler's Wife – a book that was eventually made into a movie. In the story, Henry DeTamble works as a librarian in Chicago and his future wife Clare walks up to him and says, "Henry. I'm Clare Abshire. We're going to become married to each other so I think we should talk." It turns out that Henry has a fictitious malady called Chromosome Displacement Disorder that results in Henry's bouncing around in time. After Clare and he start dating, his disorder causes him to visit Clare over one hundred fifty times while she is growing up.

At one point in the story, Henry travels back in time to visit Clare while she is in high school, and I immediately thought that would be like my traveling back in time to visit Alicia when we dated in high school. It is a good feeling to recall the first love of your life.

I kept reading and turned the page and was hit over the head emotionally with a baseball bat. There on the very next page, the story explained that Clare's sister was named Alicia. Whoa! I mean I had just thought about traveling in time to visit Alicia, and it turns out the Clare's sister's name is Alicia. I thought, "What in the world is going on here?"

About the same time, one of Alicia's friends recommended she visit a Fortune Teller. So, she went to a house run by 'Dorothea' – fortune teller extraordinaire. Dorothea talks with Alicia and senses something. All of a sudden, she says out loud, "Alicia – you're going to get back together with someone this summer who's from your past. I think it's at a birthday party or something like that."

Alicia proceeded to say, "Huh? What are you talking about? I don't know of any birthday party this summer."

Dorothea responded with more, "Well, there's some celebration that you're planning on attending soon, and you'll be meeting someone you know again. I can sense it. And, he's someone that you'll leave your husband to be with."

Alicia said, "Well, the only celebration I know of is our 45th high school reunion."

I got a call out of the blue in mid-June 2006 from Bob Wylly. He was a classmate in high school and knew both Alicia and me. He proceeded to ask me, "We're planning a 45th high school reunion on September 26 and wondered if you could make it." I told him I would be delighted to attend and proceeded to look into flights.

Bob told me he had set up a Yahoo Group for the class with photos, a database of classmates with their contact information and stories from the past. He sent me an invite to the Yahoo Group, and I logged on and looked around. I saw photos of many of the classmates and stories on what had happened to them over the years.

I then clicked on the database and saw a search field. "Hmm," I thought, "I wonder if Alicia's in there?" I entered her name, and two Alicia's came up on the screen: there were two of them in our graduating class. She was listed first, and I look to see if she was married, and sure enough, it shows her married name with maiden name in parenthesis along with her address and email address.

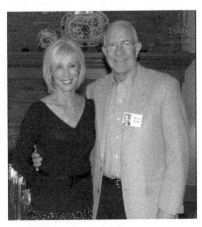

Figure 3-2 –Alicia and Gerry
Northside High School 45th reunion, September 26, 2006.

At that point, I simply stared at the entry on the screen. "Oh my god," I thought to myself. "What the hell is going on here?" I just read about Alicia in <u>Time Traveler's Wife</u> and now I find her in the Northside High School Yahoo Group. What should I do?"

I sat there and thought about it for a few minutes and then decided to write her an email. I was careful to be polite, respectful and not too forward or flirty. After all, she had felt we both needed to grow up when we had graduated from high school. She might not even reply.

After writing an appropriate but friendly email asking how she was doing after all these years, I concluded with an inquiry to see if she was planning to go to the 45th high school reunion. Off it went, with me wondering if that would be the end of it.

Alicia checked her mail and saw an email from the guy she dated in high school. "It was really unbelievable to hear from Gerry. He was being his same old way of being polite and respectful." Then she reads more, "Are you going to the Northside 45th High School Reunion?"

Bam! It's one of those long, drawn out thoughts, "Oh … my … god! This is what Dorothea was talking about in that Fortune Telling meeting. It is not a birthday party but the 45th high school reunion. And, that's who she was talking about – Gerry Purdy – the guy I dated for two years in high school. Now, he's asking me if I'm going to attend the reunion. What in the world is going on here? God, it was nice hearing from him." So, she composes a nice reply and says, yes, she will be glad to go to the reunion.

When the reply came back, I immediately thought before I read the email if she would say something like, "Thanks for your email, but I'm not going to the high school reunion and I don't want to communicate further with you. Have a good life." I almost hesitated before opening the email response. I would be devastated, as I had been 45 years ago.

So, I read the reply and was pleased to see that she was glad to have heard from me, would be happy to go to the high school reunion and, if I came in to Atlanta a day or two early, perhaps we could have dinner and get caught up on old times.

Well, right then and there, I think I began to perspire and took a big gulp of a swallow. This was a friendly and very nice email from the first girl in whom I had fallen in love. And, she's inviting me out to dinner.

Were these just coincidences? Perhaps, but the connectives and timing were certainly out of the ordinary.

We attended the 45th high school reunion in September 2006. Our relationship quickly blossomed after that because we had previously already gotten to know each other and realized that we had common values. We didn't have to take the usual time to get to know each other.

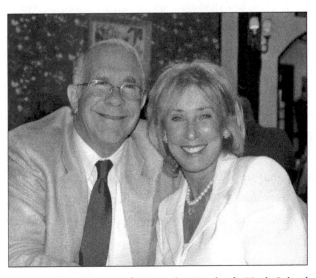

Figure 3-2 –Alicia and Gerry the Northside High School 45th reunion, September 26, 2006.

In March 2007, I proposed to Alicia on the lawn of the J. W. Marriott Ihilani Resort in Ko Olina on Oahu in Hawaii at sunset. I arranged for a guitarist to play music for us while we had a special bottle of Cristal Champagne and dinner in our own personal tent.

We got married at The Buckhead Club on October 4, 2008 with 100 friends and family. Everyone loved the shrimp and grits and the sushi stations as well as the truly great music performed by the Crystal Clear band. We then went off on our honeymoon at the Four Seasons on Nevis in the Caribbean. We were really making up for lost time.

We began living a charmed life with Alicia riding her horse most days and me taking a break from work to take a video of her riding which we then replayed at night on our large TV. We are very fortunate to have two homes – one in the Atlanta area and another in Wellington, Florida where Alicia rides in the Winter Equestrian Festival in the Hunter Division over 2' 6" jumps.

We were coming up on our third anniversary on October 4, 2011. We were going to celebrate at the Grove Park Inn in Ashville, North Carolina. We had made the reservations. It was going to be the best anniversary yet. Or, at least I thought that is the way things were going to play out.

However, everything changed on August 23, 2011.

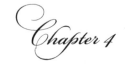

Chapter 4

STROKE DAY: AUGUST 23, 2011

"I would love to fix it all for you ... We all got bruises."

Train featuring Ashley Monroe, *Bruises*
Reprinted by permission.

I am fortunate to work out of our house. Alicia and I literally spend most of every day with each other. When she goes to ride her horse, I go along primarily to take a video of the lesson with the trainer and take a break from my working on the computer. Later, we take the dogs for a walk in the late afternoon and spend the evenings having dinner and watching some TV or a movie together.

As an industry analyst, I spend most days writing early from 6-9 am, spending some time with Alicia and then fielding calls from vendors in thirty to forty five minute briefings (some of them really are not very brief). I must do between 200 and 300 of them every year to keep up with what is going on in the mobile and wireless industry. Vendors tell me what they are doing and explain the product or service they are announcing. I listen and then ask questions. I repeat this sometimes three to five times a day.

I really do not spend much time away from home in meetings. I typically will schedule a breakfast meeting early before Alicia gets up or have a meeting in the afternoon after she is done riding. I try to schedule no more than one meeting a day out of the house.

However, on Tuesday, August 23, 2011 I had a particularly demanding day. I had actually scheduled four meetings out of the house between noon and 5:00 pm. I never can really tell from one day to the next or one week to the next how many calls or meetings I am going to have. But, on August 23, I found it almost uncomfortable that I was going to have four meetings back to back out of the house.

I did my writing, as usual in the morning. Then, Alicia and I had an appointment at Wells Fargo to sign some documents. It did not take long but we both had to be there.

After the meeting at the bank, I did a briefing call with a car rental company. They were announcing a new mobile initiative in which new systems would be rolled out in their cars that facilitated check-out and check-in using Wi-Fi placed in the car and the rental service area.

I then had a call with a business associate about the work he was doing for FitnessTrax, a company I had started to provide personalized running training programs called RunningTrax. The RunningTrax system is based on my Ph.D. thesis at Stanford. This call lasted 30 minutes. I told Alicia I was heading out to go over to have lunch with a couple of people at AT&T in their offices near Lenox Square.

From there, I had a meeting to review some design issues for RunningTrax. I called Alicia. She was doing some painting in the house – oil painting, not painting the walls (smile). Everything seemed normal. I told her I still had one more meeting to attend and that I would likely get home around 6:30 pm.

After meeting with the RunningTrax web design firm, I drove to meet someone to discuss their using RunningTrax in their marathon race.

After I finished that meeting, I called Alicia a little before 6:00 pm to tell her I was leaving the mid-town area in Atlanta and was on the way home. Since it was rather late, I suggested that I pick up dinner at Outback and bring it home. She said that would be fine. She said she would go out on to the back porch.

I called Outback and placed an order to go. We love their filet mignon dinner. Alicia has them slice her filet and place it over a salad with Blue Cheese dressing. I like mine "straight" with a salad with honey mustard.

I then drove from mid-town to Outback to pick up dinner. I called Alicia again around 6:30 pm saying that I had picked up dinner and would be home in about 15 minutes. I did not notice anything out of the ordinary – no slurred speech, no confused thoughts, nothing that would indicate anything was wrong. She sounded normal and said she was likely going to feed the dogs and get a glass of wine.

6:30 pm

It was around 6:30 pm that a clot that formed inside Alicia evidently detached from the wall of her heart, traveled up the right carotid artery and made a right hand turn into the Medial Carotid Artery (MCA). It traveled as far as it could but finally became too large to travel through the smaller arteries that branch off the MCA.

Alicia remembers my calling her to say I was on the way home. She recalled what happened next: "I remember talking to Gerry and being able to talk about his bringing dinner home. I told him I'd get up and go fix the dogs and the cat their dinner. He said that would be fine so we could sit down when he got home and have dinner. But, when I hung up talking with him, I realized that I couldn't get up. I couldn't figure out what was wrong with me. I thought this was impossible. What's causing me to not be able to get up? Are my legs cramping and preventing me from getting up?

"I sat there for 15 minutes trying different things in order to get myself moving. Nothing seemed to work. I wasn't in panic mode because there wasn't any pain. I didn't think that anything was seriously wrong. I remember telling myself, 'OK, you can do this. On the count of three, let's just get up. One … two … three.' Nothing happened. Again, I thought, 'What in the world is wrong with me? It's like I've become paralyzed. I was moving just fine a few minutes ago. I'll just have to wait until Gerry gets home, and he can help me get up and everything will be just fine.'"

6:45 pm

When I walked in the door from the garage, I immediately said, "Hi honey, I'm home." But, I didn't hear anything so I walked through the kitchen looking for Alicia. I had just talked with her on the phone on the way home.

I put the dinner I had gotten at Outback on the counter and proceeded to the family room. I went through the family room and saw her sitting on the outdoor sofa. She loves to sit out there when the weather is nice, to read and listen to the water fountain and the sounds from the outdoors.

I remember thinking that is the reason she could not hear me when I called out when I entered the house from the garage. I thought she was most likely on the back porch talking to one of her friends.

I opened the door and repeated 'Hi Honey." I could see her sitting on the outdoor sofa on the back porch. However, she did not say anything or turn toward me or react in any way. I was not alarmed for a few seconds because I thought she might have been holding her iPhone with her right hand to her right ear and might have been concentrating on the conversation. Strange. She was sitting up normally but not moving.

She did not respond when I said her name, and I thought, "What is going on here?"

I came over to the sofa and realized she was in a daze. I asked her if she was okay, and she just mumbled. Within just a few seconds, I realized something was not right. She did not react like normal. "What's wrong?" I thought. I wasn't alarmed at this point, but was more focused on finding out exactly what was wrong. I approached her and she did not turn her head and look at me.

My emotional level began to rise. My heart rate picked up and I became anxious. I remember asking her, "Alicia, what's wrong?" All I got back was a moan – it sounded like someone who could not talk like "Uhhhhh".

I thought. "This isn't good." Half of me said I simply needed to help her snap out of whatever was the problem. "Are you in pain?" I asked, as she did not appear to show any signs of pain either audibly or via movement. But, she was sitting on the sofa and was not unconscious. She responded very softly like in a whisper "Noooooo."

What struck me at that instant was that I did not have a clue what was going on or what had happened. I had never witnessed someone acting like this before. I thought, "Well, she's not having a heart attack. That's painful and the person can either report the pain or are unconscious." It was like she was in stupor.

I remember that I lightly slapped her on the face – not like being mad or angry but like in, "C'mon, Alicia, wake up!" But, she didn't respond.

At this point, I knew we had a serious, perhaps life threatening situation. I wasn't sure what was wrong. Half of me wanted to leave her and go search on the internet about her symptoms, but the stronger feeling was to stay with her and try to help her.

Before I called anyone, I tried to lift her up. I told her I was going to take her to the emergency room at Northside Hospital, and she mumbled rather softly, "Ohhhhhh Kaaaaaay." But, she could not stay balanced when I lifted her up. It was like lifting a sack of potatoes in a big sack where parts of it fell over my arms and threw me off balance.

I was frantic at this point. I knew that speed was critical to getting help – whatever the problem happened to be. I also remember thinking that I was not panicked like I would be if I came upon someone in a car accident who was bleeding and yelling. I knew that Alicia was not dead and was not unconscious. I thought that perhaps whatever is wrong could be fixed at the emergency room.

It was at that instant, when I put her down, that I realized that I had to get professional help. I debated calling 911 but thought that perhaps a quick call to our friend, Dr. David Debose, a concierge physician, might give me a rough diagnosis based on her symptoms. I was desperately trying to find a solution so the problem would go away.

I called David. He answered, and I explained to him how I found Alicia on the back porch and the symptoms of her unable to talk and move. He immediately told me that it was most likely a neurologic problem and to call 911 and get her to the emergency room right away.

All of a sudden, right there and then, I realized that Alicia was having a stroke. I knew this was serious, and I immediately realized that this was a life changing event. I did not know if she would be paralyzed for the rest of her life or be able to recover. Funny, but I thought, "Well, she's never going to be able to ride again." I believe I thought this because I could see that she had been affected and did not think it was something in which you would go to the emergency room, they would do something and you would go home.

7:00 pm

I hung up and dialed 911. I told the person who answered that I believed my wife had just had a stroke. They said they would get an ambulance there quickly. They told me to go unlock the front door. I told them that we lived in a gated community and gave them the gate pass code.

I told Alicia that I had to go unlock the front door. I ran and unlocked the front door and went back to Alicia and told her the ambulance would be there in just a few minutes. Again, she said, "Ohhhhhh Kaaaaaay." I also told her I loved her with all my heart and that we were going to get her the best help. I reassured her that we would get through this.

7:10 pm

I realized that it would be 4-6 minutes before the ambulance showed up so I quickly called Alicia's brother Bruce Grant and told him that I believed Alicia had just had a stroke, and we were going to take her to Northside Hospital. I asked if he could meet us there, and he said he would meet us at the hospital.

I began to hear the wails of the ambulance siren in the distance clearly coming down Peachtree Dunwoody Road. I thought, "Hurry up will you!" I then heard them turn in to our development, and I told Alicia, "The ambulance is here."

I got up and went to the front door and opened it up. The medics were getting out of the ambulance, and I told them that I thought that my wife had suffered a stroke. They got the stretcher out and wheeled it into the house, through the living room, and out to the back porch.

They quickly took over and said they would transport her to Northside Hospital. One of the emergency techs called Northside to say they were inbound with a likely stoke victim. It was a very busy short time. I remember that a fire truck and crew had pulled up to the house and were trying to help also.

At this point, I had to get out of the way and think for just a few seconds about what I needed to take to the hospital. I told the driver that I would get Alicia's wallet that had her identity and insurance cards.

We had a dog and a cat. I made sure they got out of the way from all the commotion, but I did not have time to feed them. They had water so I knew they could get by for a few hours.

7:15 pm

As we all migrated to the ambulance, I thought about whom I needed to call. They told me to sit in the front of the ambulance. There was someone in the back with Alicia. They had put an oxygen mask over her face. I thought that the first three people I need to call were her children. Since her son Grant lived nearby in Decatur, I called him and explained to him what had happened and told him to meet us at Northside Hospital.

I then called her daughter Sandy. I am still a bit amazed that I reached Grant and Sandy on the first try. I told them that their mom had suffered a stroke and that I would call again once we knew a bit more about the situation.

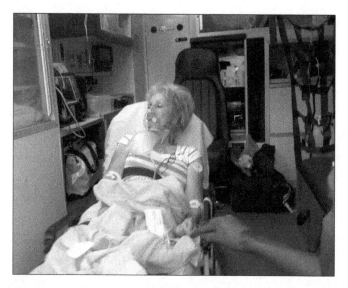

Figure 4-1. Alicia arriving at Northside Hospital at 7:22 pm.

I thought, "OK, I have informed her kids, and because she has so many close friends, I need to call a few of them. The siren was blazing and we were on Peachtree-Dunwoody Road racing to the hospital.

I called Mary Portman, Kathy Sands, Linda Keefe and Lynn Ford. I had to leave a message for Kathy but got the others live. Mary and Linda said they would come to the hospital. We were pulling into the hospital and knew I had to give my attention to Alicia and be there for the initial assessment. I had many others to call but they would have to wait. We arrived at the hospital at 7:22 pm (Figure 4-1).

They wheeled Alicia into a room and the nurse and Phil Harris, M.D., attending emergency Room physician, made a quick assessment. It was really horrible because Alicia could not talk other than a weak mumble and could not move. They agreed she likely had suffered a stroke. They asked what time it occurred, and I told them that I had talked with her around 6:30 pm and said I was on the way home and got there fifteen minutes later and found her unable to move or talk at 6:50 pm.

They explained that they needed to determine if the stroke was ischemic (clot) or hemorrhage bleeding and they needed to do a quick CT scan.

7:45 pm

Alicia was wheeled "stat" (emergency) to the CT scanner. I had to wait for her to get back. Mary Portman and her friend Jim Adams showed up as did Lynn and Alan Ford, who lived close by. I met them all in the lobby area after the nurse told me that she would come to get me as soon as they brought Alicia back from the CT scan.

Alicia's son Grant came in about the same time as Linda. I wanted Linda there because her husband had experienced a stroke years before. He remained quite debilitated partially paralyzed for the rest of his life. She knew what was going on and almost immediately told me that I should get Alicia to the Marcus Stroke Center at Grady Hospital. I then remembered the billboards that Grady had around town with the slogan, "There's one word for stroke: Grady." But, I could not make that happen until she came back from having the CT scan.

Mary Portman then called a mutual good friend, Matt Burrell, MD. He was able to come immediately to the hospital to help interact with the family about Alicia's condition.

8:15 pm

The nurse then came and told me that Alicia was back from getting the CT scan. We returned to Alicia's room in the emergency room area and met Dr. Gerald Silverboard, attending neurologist. The check for hemorrhaging was negative and so they told Alicia and me that they were going to administer tissue plasminogen activator (tPA) often called "clot buster," the first treatment process for those with an ischemic stroke. This was administered at 8:25 pm or a little less than two hours after the onset of the stroke.

It was going to take thirty to forty-five minutes to determine to what degree the tPA would be successful. I made a few more calls.

At this point, we had Mary, Jim, Bruce and Dr. Matt Burrell all in the room. They administered the tPA via an IV. After a few minutes, you could see the tPA starting to work. It was very exciting and hopeful to see some of the symptoms go away. Alicia could move her left leg and arm but not her fingers. She started to enunciate some words, but she was clearly still compromised.

10:00 pm

There was a lot of conferring on the status between the attending ER doctor, the attending neurologist Dr. Silverboard and Dr. Burrell. Dr. Silverboard wanted to find if out there was a clot and where it was located, so he ordered an MRI at around 10 pm. Dr. Burrell talked very re-assuredly and slowly with Alicia to explain why they were doing the MRI. She seemed to understand, I gave her a kiss. Off she went again.

We all relocated to the lobby as could be an hour before she was back from the MRI. I remember that I used Alicia's iPhone to call family and friends, mostly because all of her friend's phone numbers were in her phone.

I called Connie Blythe who was a long-time riding friend of Alicia's. This was Tuesday, and we were scheduled to leave on Thursday for The DeBordieu Club in Georgetown, SC to attend Connie and Frank's son's wedding. We could communicate only via voice mail as there wasn't very good coverage there at the resort. She took care of canceling our reservations even though she had more challenging things to worry about. Hurricane Irene was bearing down on the South Carolina coast and could cause many plans including relocating the outdoor rehearsal dinner.

I called long-time friends Eleanor Effinger and Kathy Sands and gave them an update. I called Alicia's daughter Sandy to keep her informed. I felt very upset at this point. I didn't know what was going to happen to Alicia. My mind was buzzing, trying to make sure that all of her friends were notified. I was worried I was going to forget one of Alicia's close friends. They all loved Alicia and any of them would be really upset if I did not inform them of the situation. Calls went out to Peggy Knight, Wendy Gifford, Susan Traynor, Kathy Whiteside and Barbara Goldsmith – all riding friends. I kept thinking, "Who have I missed? Oh dear, I forgot to call Lynn Schroeder and Lavonne Hampton." I found myself struggling to remember who needed to be called.

Alicia's daughter Sandy wanted to jump on a plane, but I told her to hold off just a bit until we knew what was going to happen. Linda Keefe recommended I get Alicia to the Marcus Stroke Center, but I could not consider doing that until she came back from the MRI test.

I sat in the waiting room area with Alicia's brother Bruce, Mary Portman, Lynn and Alan Ford, Alicia's son Grant and Linda Keefe. We talked about options, I had an image of dealing with Alicia being partially paralyzed for the rest of her life. I had seen Linda's husband for years suffering from afflictions caused by a major stroke, and I suddenly broke down. I started to cry and felt embarrassed a bit in front of all these friends. I completely "lost it" and felt helpless that there was not anything that I could do to help Alicia. Ever since we got together, I felt it was my job to take care of her, to be the person she could rely on always to be there and to help her deal with major problems.

I remembered that when Alicia and I were in Hawaii in March 2007 on the way to Japan, I had made arrangements to propose to Alicia at sunset. I called Bruce to ask him for permission to marry his sister. Alicia's dad, who was CEO of Plantation Pipeline Corp. in Atlanta, had died suddenly of a heart attack at age 56 when Alicia was a sophomore at the University of Georgia. I thought that since I could not call her dad, I would do the next best thing and call Bruce. I told him that I loved Alicia with all my heart, that I would take good care of her and with their dad no longer living, I wanted his permission to marry Alicia. He said, "Hey, hey … I'd be honored if you'd marry Alicia." He told me it he would appreciate it very much if I would take the responsibilities of his sister off his hands. We laughed a bit about it. I remember him as always being very nice to me when Alicia and I dated in high school, and I feel that Bruce is a brother of mine today.

I talked with Lynn Ford and Grant as Lynn's children and Grant grew up together and were life-long friends. Lynn sat there and told me how wonderful Alicia was and that she would come out of this OK. Lynn is that kind of person who is always bringing sunshine into everyone's life.

I talked with Linda about options since she had experience dealing with her husband's stroke. She felt was distraught over her husband and

Alicia was being afflicted with a stroke. But, she was practical and I wanted her counsel. We both agreed that we would make arrangements to transfer Alicia to the Marcus Stroke Center unless something else came back from the MRI.

Mary Portman is wonder woman. She juggles the demands of being a well-known personality in Atlanta yet she is also deeply spiritual. We have had many long conversations – Alicia, Mary and me – about consciousness, Mary feels we are all interconnected. She can understand and appreciate what many people would consider "strange things" like the premonition from the fortune teller who told Alicia she was going to get together with someone at a birthday party.

Just before Alicia left to have the MRI test done, Mary did some really cute things: she took off Alicia's wedding ring and heart necklace. She said she would keep them in a safe place until Alicia got back home. She put the rings in her purse and wore the heart necklace. She said, "I'll wear it until Alicia feels better. That way it will be safe." She could not pass up wearing that necklace. She loved it ever since I bought it for Alicia for Christmas in 2006.

Since Alicia was still having the MRI test completed, I called a number of other friends. I went through Alicia's contacts to do a cross reference as I did not want to hear from any one of them that I did not let them know. I called Nina MacRae, Sherri Crawford and tried to reach Connie Blythe again and left her an update.

11:00 pm

The nurse came out and told us Alicia was back from the MRI. We all traipsed back into the emergency room. It felt like there were a dozen people in there. Matt went to confer with Dr. Silverboard about the results of the MRI. When they both came back, Dr. Silverboard told Alicia that the radiologist said he could not find a clot so they were not sure exactly what to do other than check her into a Northside patient room and see how she responded to the tPA. They would start rehabilitation and see how things developed.

I think you could have heard a pin drop in the room. There was dead silence. I felt as if the carpet had been pulled out from under me. I remember becoming emotional and almost fainting. My heart was pounding like mad. "Oh No!" I thought. I looked over at Linda Keefe, and she had a tear in her eye. I could feel her all the way across the room, "No, no, this shouldn't be happening. Not again!" She started shaking her head as in "No, this is not right. You need to get her out of here!" I was holding one of Alicia's hands. She just looked at us and seemed to acknowledge that she understood what was being told to her.

I reflect back now and am glad that she was not really conscious and aware of everything yet. She was still in major compromise to her brain. She could not possibly understand what was being said or, perhaps more accurately, the life-long implications of what we were being informed. Mary was holding Alicia's other hand. The emotions were swelling up in everyone's heart, throat and eyes. It was like she had been told that she was about to die and everyone should prepare for that outcome, including her.

As this discussion was going on while we were all in a state of very sad and upset emotions, a nurse came in and told Dr. Silverboard that the radiologist needed to talk with him ASAP. He left along with Dr. Burrell. We all just looked at each other. Imagine what this scene was like: Alicia – bless her heart – was lying on the bed barely able to move. She looked ragged. Mary, Linda, Grant, Bruce and I were all looking at each other like the person we all loved was almost gone. She was not dead, but she was never going to be the same – somewhere between a paralyzed vegetable and, perhaps, someone who can barely walk, limping with half her face paralyzed as in the classic stroke scenario. I could tell that everyone was thinking the same thing.

I know that I felt angry at this point. I thought "Hey, this isn't fair. She's the most wonderful person in the entire world. She gives so much love and counsel to others. She is healthy – God, she is about the healthiest person I know for her age. How in hell could she be the one lying here with a life-threatening stroke? It seemed more likely that I would be lying there rather than her. I felt as my life with Alicia was being taken away from me. Why was such a bad thing happening to such a good person? It's not fair. It's absolutely, positively not fair!" No one said anything. It was like every one suddenly went from talking to being silent and sending non-verbal emotions to each other. It felt as if we were in suspended animation for what seemed like ten minutes. Realistically, it was just a couple of minutes.

The spell was broken as Dr. Silverboard and Dr. Burrell came back into the room. All eyes suddenly flashed to Dr. Silverboard who said to Alicia, "Well, I've just had a follow up call from the radiologist. He re-looked at the MRI, and he definitely sees a clot in the base of your brain. It's conclusive. I recommend that you be transferred to the Marcus Stroke Center at Grady Hospital as soon as possible. I'm going to call and notify them that you're coming." He did not wait to field questions from us as he felt it was important to notify Grady ASAP. He just turned and walked out of the room.

Right then and there, Linda said, "Finally, we're getting her the help she needs. I've been telling you for the past two hours to get her out of here." Dr. Burrell talked to Alicia and all of us in the room, "This really changes everything. Grady has one of the best stroke centers in the country. Since the radiologist has found a clot, it is best we get you transported there so they can determine the best way to deal with it."

The emotions in the room went from total despair to cautious optimism. It was like someone had come in the room and said, "Wait! She's not going to die! She's going to live!" The atmosphere in the room was once again very emotional. I immediately thought, "What does this mean? What can they do to help?"

Dr. Silverboard came back and said, "I've talked with Dr. Raul Nogueira, chief of neurosurgery at Grady. He wants the MRI and Alicia to get there ASAP. I've put in orders to get an ambulance and I'll get the MRI ready to go with her."

At that point – literally – my phone rang. I said, "Hello, this is Gerry" but not sure who was calling.

"This is Dr. Nogueira at Grady. Dr. Silverboard explained to me the condition of your wife and that they can see a clot at the base of your wife's brain. I want you to get her here absolutely as soon as possible. I am going to try to remove the clot, and if I can do that, she'll have a chance at a full recovery."

I thanked him and said we would get there in the next half hour. I remember my throat filling up and I almost lost it right then and there. "Full recovery" rang out in my head. Just a few minutes prior, we had all felt she was just about gone or going to be a paralyzed for the rest of her life, and now he's saying "full recovery." This is too much to grasp.

I got off the phone and told everyone what Dr. Nogueira had told me. I looked around the room and everyone – except perhaps Alicia – was standing there with their mouths wide open as in "I don't believe this." It was like one of those scenes in a TV show or movie where the wide mouth opened look was frozen and the camera went around the periphery showing everyone in stop action.

I was very emotional as I took Alicia's hand and told her that we were going to take her to Grady and the surgeon there felt he could likely remove the clot that had caused the stroke. "Ohhhhh kaaaay." It hurt me to my core to hear her respond like this. However, I now believed we might be able to have a positive outcome.

The next moment was like right after the general says, "OK, let's go!" Everyone started to mobilize. I said I needed to go home briefly to feed the dogs, get my medications and my car. Linda Keefe said she would take me. Grant said he would drive my car to Grady so I could have one to drive home later. He would get a friend to pick him up at the hospital. I asked the ER nurse the ETA for the ambulance. She said it would be there in about ten minutes.

11:30 pm

Mary, Bruce and the Ford family decided to go home. I promised to give them a call or text them with an update once we got to Grady and knew more. We lived only one mile from Northside Hospital, so Linda took me to the house so I could take care of a few things and get my car.

When I entered the house, I noticed the cold filet minion from Outback sitting on the counter where I had briefly put it down when I had come home five hours earlier. I told Fritzie, our dachshund dog, "Fritzie, how about some filet mignon for dinner?" She took one whiff and started to wag her tale. I mixed that in with her kibble. She was one happy dog. I gave some cat kibble to Angel our white cat. I got my medicines for the next twenty four hours and put them in my pocket, took Fritzie out to the bathroom, got in my car and was back at Northside in about ten minutes total. The ambulance had just pulled in and the attendants were taking a wheeled stretcher inside. I asked them if they were there to take a patient to Grady and they affirmed that was their task.

We went in and got Alicia's clothes in that little plastic bag that they give you when you check in to a hospital emergency room or for outpatient surgery. I found Dr. Silverboard and thanked him for his help. I reviewed the logistics with Linda and Grant. I would go in the ambulance and Linda and Grant would caravan behind the ambulance. I kissed Alicia as the attendants got ready to move her to the mobile stretcher. "We're going to get through this. Let's get you the help you deserve."

They put Alicia in the ambulance, and I got in the front seat. The red lights went on. Once we were out on Peachtree Dunwoody Road, the sirens started blaring. We went down to Glenridge Connector and onto GA 400 south and then we really picked up steam. We were all flying down GA 400 at 80 mph with lights and sirens blazing and the caravan all in tow. It reminded me of a Presidential caravan.

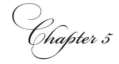

GRADY STROKE CENTER

"I had a dream so big and loud
I jumped so high I touched the clouds.
Wo-o-o-o-oh [2x]
I stretched my hands out to the sky
We danced with monsters through the night
Wo-o-o-o-oh [2x]
This is going to be the best day of my life."

American Authors, *Best Day of My Life*
Reprinted by permission.

As soon as we arrived at Grady Hospital around 12:15 am Wednesday morning, Alicia's son, Grant, and our close friend Linda and I met with Dr. Nogueira in the Marcus Stroke Center waiting area. This is where the entire story gets really interesting.

Dr. Nogueira explained that Alicia had a clot in her brain that caused the stroke. He said that if we did nothing, Alicia would likely be paralyzed for the rest of her life. I realized right then and there just how serious the situation was. Gulp.

Instead, he recommended that he do a procedure to try to remove the clot and, thus, reduce the long-term negative impact on the brain. But, he also explained there were risks in doing the procedure. I asked for the rough statistics. He explained that while every patient is different, they were able to successfully remove the clot in 93% of the cases. However, in around 7% of the cases, they either were not able to remove the clot or the situation became worse due to puncturing the artery and causing further bleeding.

I turned to Grant and told him I thought this should be a family decision. I wanted Alicia to have the best chance of having some recovery instead of being paralyzed. I know she would say, "Go for it!" Grant agreed and so did Linda. In addition, I wanted to get Alicia's daughter Sandy to concur. Sandy lives on Central Time and an hour earlier so it was not as late as it was in Atlanta.

I fortunately reached Sandy and explained to her the situation and that we had to make a very quick decision: either to do nothing with Alicia very likely paralyzed or sign the consent allowing Dr. Nogueira and his team to do the procedure to attempt to remove the clot and, thus, possibly reduce the long-term effects of the stroke. I gave her the statistics and told her there were some risks in doing the procedure. She said that her mom would want to have the procedure done and concurred with Grant and me.

Although I had legal authority to sign the consent form by myself, I asked Grant to co-sign with me. Grant and I signed then both signed the consent form. At this point, we thought we were done. I expected Dr. Nogueira to leave and go do the procedure.

However, Dr. Nogueira explained that we had to make a second decision. He said there were two devices approved by the FDA to help in the retrieval and removal of the clot and one new device that was under trial but not yet approved by the FDA.

There were two devices approved at the time by the FDA for removal of clots (called Transcatheter Embolus Retrieval): 1) an aspirator device that uses suction to withdraw the clot material and 2) a corkscrew-like device that goes through the clot and pulls it out. A newer third device called stent retriever was going through FDA approval. (It has since been approved.)

The stent retriever device works like a stent used to unclog a coronary artery. It is a small mesh-like device that is inserted in the catheter, passed through to the beginning of where the clot is lodged and then carefully pushed through in the clot in the brain artery. The mesh then expands in the clot essentially grabbing hold of it. After a short wait, the device is removed along with the portion of the clot that has become intertwined with the mesh. It works like a Roto-Rooter in reverse since the clot material that sticks to the mesh is withdrawn from the brain.

I asked Dr. Nogueira if the new device made any difference. Was it equivalent to the two devices that were approved or was it better? He explained that he had been very successful using the new stent retriever device. He said that he was just about 100% successful in withdrawing a significant amount of clot material in the cases in which he has been able to use it to date. It has helped patient's arteries in the brain "re-perfuse" or begin circulation again beyond the clot.

I distinctly remember at that point saying to Dr. Nogueira, "Well, if that's the case, please use the stent retriever device." I thought we were done again. But, Dr. Nogueira responded that it was not that easy. He explained that since the stent retriever device was under FDA review, the use of it was completely randomized to make the results objective and not biased by the patients that the neurosurgeon felt would have the best outcome.

Dr. Nogueira said he had no control over whether he could use stent retriever or not. I asked him how it was decided whether to use it or not. He explained that it was like having an envelope that was opened once the procedure started which told him whether to user stent retriever or not.

"Wait a minute," I exclaimed. "This is my wife and childhood sweetheart in there. Who do I need to call to ensure that you'll be able to use the stent retriever device?" I thought I would call the White House if necessary. "Random" was OK for medical trials, but since it clearly worked better than the other two devices, I wanted Dr. Nogueira to use it and not the other devices that did not have as positive an outcome.

He explained that there was no one I could call. Even the President couldn't over-ride the random trial. I was a bit upset, stressed and not sure what to do.

I was quite emotional at this point and likely a bit irrational. I asked Dr. Nogueira, "Before you go in there, can you tell me what qualifications you have to do this procedure?" Grant Mitchell looked at me with an expression of disbelief. He later said that he had thought, "Are you crazy? He's a neurosurgeon, and you're asking him if he's qualified?" I had to admit in reflection that it was an unreasonable question but I cared so much for Alicia that I wanted to be sure the doctor was qualified.

Dr. Nogueira replied, "Well," he said, "I was head of Neurosurgery at Mass General Hospital for over ten years and then relocated to the Marcus Stroke Center within the past couple of years. And, I'm the principal investigator in the US for the stent retriever device."

Instantly, my brain went from a totally emotional inquisition to thinking, "OK, why are you still sitting here? Get in there and get that damn clot out of my wife's brain!" When you are very emotional at times like this, it is hard to think clearly.

Grant and I signed the consent to be included in the FDA trial. That gave us at least a fighting chance that he would get the approval to use the stent retriever device in the Operating Room.

Dr. Nogueira took the forms. As he left to go back into surgery, he explained, "I'll do my best to help your wife. But, realize that this is a rather lengthy procedure. I will be in there for three to four hours. I'll come out when I'm done and let you know how it went." Off he walked in his scrub attire toward the Marcus Stroke Center operating room.

Grant, Linda and I stood there looking at each other a little bit like, "OK, what do we do now?" Linda said that she was going to go home. Grant had driven my car to Grady and said he had a friend who was going to pick him up.

I was not going anywhere. I knew that the Alicia's life lay in the hands of Dr. Raul Nogueira. I was going to sit there in the waiting room until he came out and let me know how the procedure went.

My Time during the Surgery

When Dr. Nogueira left the waiting room to go to the OR to do the procedure on Alicia, I sat alone in this very quiet waiting room with nothing to do. They did not have a TV. It was simply a room with chairs and a desk for the receptionist who was only there during the daytime. There was not anyone in there the entire time I was waiting for Dr. Nogueira to finish the procedure. I did not have either a pen or paper. The feeling was one of being helpless with an ardent desire to have Alicia make a full recovery and not become paralyzed for the rest of her life. She is such a beautiful person that so many people loved.

My first thought was that if the procedure was not successful, her normal life would be over. I was really scared that our wonderful relationship would change into one in which I was simply a caretaker of a paralyzed person. I quietly prayed that the doctors and support staff would do everything they possibly could do to help Alicia have a positive outcome.

As part of our getting back together, we decided to have a glass of champagne before dinner each night to toast the good things that happened during the day. We had our toast the previous night celebrating good things that were happening in our lives and the lives around us. It simply was not time to end this very special love story and all of our traditions. You hear so many people talk about how precious life is and how it can all disappear in a wink of an eye. I sat there very afraid and not sure what to do.

I then got two calls between 2:00 and 3:00 am while Alicia was in surgery. One was from Alicia's friend Eleanor Effinger who was home but very concerned about one of the closest friends she had in the world. She asked me if I would like her to come down to Grady Hospital and sit with me. I told her that it would not be very productive at this point since Alicia was in surgery, and we really would not know anything for a few hours. I promised to call her once I knew how the procedure went.

The other call was from Kathy Sands, another of Alicia's close friends whom she has known for over thirty years since their children were young. Kathy would do anything for anybody. She is truly one of God's gifts for kindness. She also asked if she should come over to the hospital. I told her that there was nothing to do but sit and wait until the procedure was over. I promised that I would call her when I heard something definite.

I had some thoughts about Alicia that I wanted to record as they popped into my head during the long wait. I scrounged around and found a small pencil in the receptionist's desk drawer and finally found some small sheets of paper that the receptionist used for notes to give patient's family and friends during the day. I sat down at the reception desk and began writing my thoughts as they came to my mind.

I sat there over the course of three hours and wrote an 11-page letter to Alicia to document the events and to let her know how much I loved her. I read this letter over and over partly to edit it and partly to reinforce my hope for a positive outcome.

The Procedure

Dr. Nogueira used a process called Transcatheter Embolus Retrieval or Endarectomy. Here's a brief summary of the process he used along with some visuals taken in the OR during the procedure.

It turns out that Dr. Nogueira was given approval to use the stent retriever device in the procedure. I did not know this until he came out of surgery at 4:19 am, but you'll see the stent retriever device in a later photo. I am sure he was pleased to use the device since he has had such good success with it in the past.

To begin, Dr. Nogueira inserted a catheter in Alicia's leg - similar to the procedure to do a heart catheterization, only he takes the catheter up into the right carotid artery that comes off the main artery leaving the heart. You can see this in Figure 5-1 where the catheter traveled once it was inserted in the artery in Alicia's leg and moved vertically toward the heart.

The catheter traveled up through the Descending Aorta past the Left Subclavian Artery and Left Common Artery to the Brachiocephalic Artery. It was like traveling through an Italian city with roundabouts: "Go North and then take the third right in the roundabout." Once in the Brachiocephalic artery, he "stayed right" to go up the Right Common Carotid Artery.

This placed the catheter at the Right Carotid Artery at the base of the brain. At this point, he inserted some dye that would show up on an X-ray. This lit up the areas further up the Right Carotid Artery. The location of the clot could be identified when the dye stopped flowing.

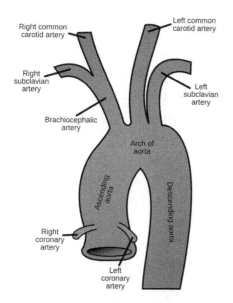

Figure 5-1. Anatomy of the aorta and location of the right carotid artery. The catheter was inserted in Alicia's leg artery and passed up through the descending aorta and right up the brachiocephalic artery and right again up the right common carotid artery.

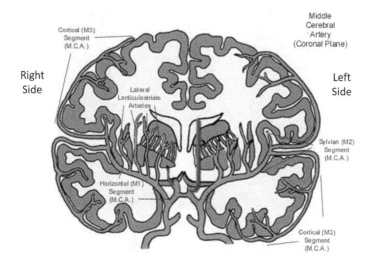

Figure 5-2. The anatomy of the right and left coronary arteries. The Medial Cerebral Artery (MCA) travels outward from the center of the brain with small Lateral Lenticulostriate Arteries and then on to feed blood to the rest of the brain.

Figure 5-2 shows the anatomy of the areas that travel off the Right Coronary Artery.

Figure 5-3 shows first image taken during the procedure to remove the clot that was causing Alicia's stroke. Dye was injected through the catheter. An image is captured by an angiogram – an X-ray test that uses fluoroscopy to take pictures of the blood flow within an artery (such as the aorta). The dye worked its way up through the right side of the brain. Dye was not put in the Left Carotid Artery so that area doesn't show any dark areas.

You can see the dye in the angiogram in Figure 5-3. It goes vertically up through the center of the brain. But, the dye diverts to the left in the photo and suddenly stops at the point shown by

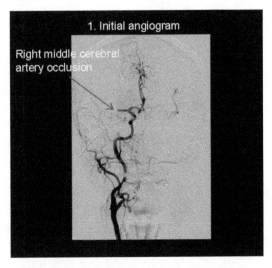

Figure 5-3. Angiogram of Alicia's left Carotid Artery with dye released. Normally, the entire left side of the image (Alicia's right brain) would be totally filled with dye showing circulation throughout the right side of the brain. But, the dye stops at the point shown by the blue arrow. The clot is located at this point because the dye suddenly stops when it should continue to travel to Alicia's right side of her brain.

the blue arrow. Normally, the dye would continue to fill out the left side of the image (right side of Alicia's head), but, instead, the dye suddenly stops. Thus, Dr. Nogueira knew at this point where the clot was located. The next task was to use the device to retrieve the clot in a "reverse Roto-Rooter" process.

Figure 5-4 shows the anatomy of the location of the clot that corresponds to the angiogram in Figure 5-3. You can see that the clot traveled up the right carotid artery and then made a left turn (to the right in Alicia's brain). It finally became lodged in the medial cerebral artery (MCA) when the artery became too small to let the clot pass further down.

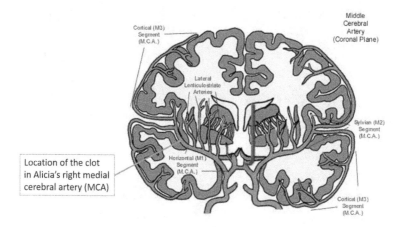

Figure 5-4. Location of the clot in Alicia's right medial cerebral artery (MCA) shown in the green circle. This is the anatomy that corresponds to the angiogram image shown in Figure 5-3.

Next, Dr. Nogueira fed the catheter up the carotid and down the MCA artery to the front edge of the clot. He inserted the stent retriever device through the catheter. The mesh-like material in the device was slowly pushed through the clot.

Dr. Nogueira told me that he feels the pressure of the clot against the catheter. He then gently pushed the stent retriever device through the clot and allowed it to expand into the clot. The mesh expands like a stent in the heart, only here, the mesh embeds itself into the clot. After a short time, he pulled the stent retriever device back out through the catheter and placed the clot material on a tray and went back to do the procedure again. You can see the catheter in the X-ray image shown in Figure 5-5.

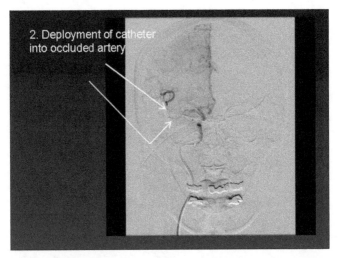

2. Deployment of catheter into occluded artery

Figure 5-5. This is an X-ray image of Alicia's head. You can see her teeth crowns near the bottom as well as an outline of her eyes. The catheter is shown coming from below up to the area which was blocked by the clot. It was at this point that Dr. Nogueira was able to use the stent retriever device to extract most of the clot.

He related that he did this process five times and extracted clot material three of the five times. Finally, the device reached the other side of the clot and blood rushed through the opened artery. The device is composed of mesh-like material. Each time he pushed the device through the clot material; the device naturally expanded into the remaining clot material and was then withdrawn.

Dr. Nogueira clearly had excellent results with the new device in this procedure to help Alicia. Take a look at the angiogram Figure 5-6 after he removed the clot. You can see the three pieces of clot material along with the stent retriever device that was used to extract the clot. The web of the stent retriever device expands into the clot and assists in gathering it so that it can be extracted through the catheter.

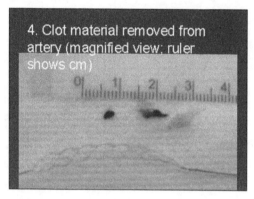

Figure 5-6. Three pieces of the blood clot are shown after they were extracted from Alicia's medial cerebral artery (MCA) using the stent retriever device as shown at the bottom part of the picture.

Dr. Nogueira took one final angiogram image of Alicia's brain as shown in Figure 5-7. It shows full circulation to Alicia's right brain after he was able to remove the clot material. This is the real "wow" image because if you compare it with the first angiogram image, the differences are striking.

At this point, the procedure was over, and Alicia was taken to the Intensive Care Unit (ICU) in the Stroke Center to rest and recover.

Dr. Nogueira came out of surgery at 4:19 am He told me he was able to use the new stent retriever device on Alicia and felt he had very good

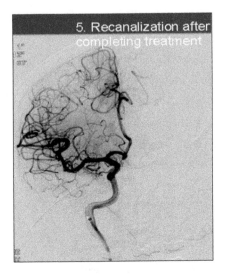

5. Recanalization after
completing treatment

Figure 5-7.
Angiogram after the
clot material was
removed from Alicia's
right cerebral artery
(MCA). Her right
brain is now getting
full circulation.

results. I literally broke down, crying with joy and appreciation. He knew it was a trying experience and put his hand on my shoulder in support and comfort.

He explained that the clot had been lodged in her Medial Cerebral Artery (MCA). He drew Alicia's condition on a pad. He showed the carotid artery and the MCA and drew a number of small lines off the MCA called the Lateral Lenticulostriate Arteries. Finally, he drew a small clogged up area just past these small branch arteries and told me that the clot had been lodged there.

Dr. Nogueira then showed me the angiogram photos on his iPhone taken in the OR: the "before" image showed the right hemisphere of her brain totally white due to no circulation, while the "after" clearly showed return to normal circulation. He said that most of the damage from the stroke was located in the small artery in the base of the brain. He explained that when a stroke happens due to a clot stopping circulation in the brain, the neurons die at the rate of one million cells a minute. Even though that meant that millions of neurons had died since the onset of the stroke, he said that because there were tens of billions of neurons in the brain and the area affected was not 100% dead, Alicia would be able to find ways to "work around" the affected areas and get back many of the functions lost due to the stroke.

He added that he felt Alicia would be able to return to full health. But, because Alicia had been through a lot of brain stress due to the clot, the reduced circulation for a number of hours and the stress of the surgery, it would take some time for her to get back to the way she was before the stroke.

He asked if I would like to see Alicia. We went into stroke intensive care unit (ICU) where she was asleep in a bed. He tried to shake her to wake her up, but she did not respond. I told him that she was a very sound sleeper and took a half an Ambien each night. I also mentioned that I thought she was quite sensitive to anesthesia as well as other medicines. He concurred that Alicia would likely be out for four to five more hours. He suggested that we both go home and get some rest and come back later. He assured me that another stroke was not likely now that he had removed the clot. I thanked him sincerely for all he did to give Alicia the opportunity to live the rest of her life and not have it taken away so suddenly and unfairly.

I quickly made two calls: one to Eleanor Effinger and another to Kathy Sands who had both stayed up all night waiting an updated status of Alicia. I told both of them the good news that the surgery was successful. I found myself choking up and unable to talk normally about it because it was so emotional. They were so wonderful to have "held a vigil" for their close friend. Until this day, I don't know how they managed to stay up all night. But, both of them were very thankful to hear that their dear friend was likely to recover.

Post Surgery
I left the hospital and went to the parking garage to get my car and drive home. Grant had told me exactly where he parked the car on the second

floor because the parking lot was totally full when he arrived around 12:15 am. I had to laugh when I came out of the elevator on the second floor and turned to see if I could find my car. "There it is," I thought giggling a bit. It was the only car left on the second floor.

I went home and found our dog Fritzie excited to see me. I fixed her a little something to eat from the filet steaks I had gotten at Outback for our dinner the previous evening. (As a side note, it has been very difficult for Alicia and me to go back to Outback since the stroke as it reminds us of the evening that the stroke happened. It was almost like thinking rather foolishly that we did not want to risk getting Outback take-out because it might cause another stroke. We do not have any problem going to dinner there now, but it was a sensitive manner for a couple of years).

It was a bit strange going to bed just before 6:00 am. I don't know how young people can party all night and be good to go the next morning. As I was getting ready to get into the bed to get a few hours of sleep, something really amazing happened that I can remember clear as day.

Each night when we go to bed, our white cat named Angel comes up on our bed and sits on Alicia's head for a while – sometime for hours but sometimes just for a few minutes. It is her way of loving her "mother." We would often say, "Come on Angel, come up on the bed and sit on mommy's pillow," to which she would jump up on the bed, walk over and place herself on Alicia's pillow resting herself against Alicia's head. She spends part of almost every night doing this.

Well, when I got in the bed, Angel jumped up and was looking over to find her mommy who was not there. I told her that her mommy was in the hospital, but she would be coming home soon. I swear to God, it was like she understood her mommy was ill. She walked over to Alicia's pillow and began to knead on it over and over. I sat that there looking at her and thinking, "Oh my God. Angel knows that something has happened to her mommy and is showing love for her by kneading on her pillow." And if that wasn't strange enough, she repeated the same activity the next three nights as a vigil until Alicia came home on Saturday, Aug. 27. Clearly, cats – and Angel in particular – have some uncanny abilities.

It took me maybe thirty seconds to fall asleep. I said a quick prayer thanking God for giving Alicia a chance to live out her life instead of her being taken away from her friends, family and loved ones. I also thanked Dr. Nogueira for his skill in being able to extract the clot.

I remember waking suddenly around 8:00 am Wednesday morning with my iPhone ringing. I realized that I should have put it on Silent before going to bed. It was Linda Keefe. She wanted to get an update on Alicia since the last time we talked was at Grady Hospital the previous evening. I told her that the procedure was successful and that Alicia was anticipated to make a complete recovery. She expressed relief and amazement. I also got a call from Mary Portman who, like Linda, didn't know what happened since the previous evening. I filled her in. She said she would come visit Alicia later in the day.

After I got off the call, I decided to get dressed and return to the hospital to check on Alicia. I knew that I would likely be exhausted later that day from not getting a full night's sleep. However, Alicia and her recovery were more important than getting another hour or two of sleep.

On the way to the hospital, I talked briefly with Alicia's daughter Sandy. She said she was on the way to visit her mom driving to Atlanta.

Back at the Hospital

When I got back to the hospital, I was escorted into Alicia's room in Intensive Care. Alicia had just awaken from the anesthesia. She was alert but still a bit groggy. I gave her a kiss. I have to admit I was shaking inside, unsure of what her condition might be. It was great to see her awake.

I met Dr. Michael Frankel, Director of the Marcus Stroke Center and Professor, Emory School of Medicine. He and his team were interacting with Alicia and beginning to do a test that would provide an assessment of Alicia's condition.

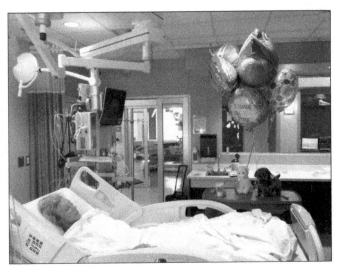

Figure 5-8. Alicia in the stroke center ICU resting on Wednesday, Aug. 24. Note the two small stuffed animals with the balloons that were sent by friends Tom and Sharron Marshall. One of them looks like our cat Angel and the other looks like our Dachshund Fritzie.

It turned out that Dr. Frankel and I have a common friend in Dr. Randy Martin, cardiologist with Piedmont Heart Institute and prior Associate Dean of the Emory Medical School. Dr. Frankel studied under Dr. Martin at Emory. In another coincidence, Alicia's daughter went to school with Dr. Martin's daughter. Dr. Frankel said he would contact Dr. Martin and notify him about Alicia's stroke and ask him to drop by to see Alicia.

Dr. Frankel and the Neurology team led by Dr. Lisa Rivera then did their first stroke assessment on Alicia following the surgical procedure.

The assessment is a combination of verbal and movement requests to see how a patient responds. It was important to form a baseline following the surgical procedure to extract the clot. I was particularly interested in this initial test because the last time I had seen Alicia awake was in the emergency room at Northside Hospital where she was partially paralyzed on the left side. While tPA had gotten Alicia to the point that she could move, she still could not lift her left arm, her fingers on her left hand or her left leg.

Alicia was a little slow but seemed aware and basically was the same "person" she was before the stroke. I was thrilled to see her "back" but unsure how much damage the stroke had caused while the clot was in place in the lower part of her brain.

Dr. Rivera asked her to move her left arm. I froze. She simply lifted her left arm – almost like nothing had ever happened. I had tears in my eyes. I could not believe it. Here Alicia was paralyzed twelve hours earlier and now, following surgery to remove the clot, she had regained the ability to lift her left arm.

Dr. Rivera next asked Alicia to wiggle her fingers. She wiggled them. She could not do that the previous night at Northside Hospital. Dr. Rivera asked her to touch her nose. She touched her nose. She asked Alicia to lift/move her left leg. She did that, too. Dr. Rivera asked her to smile, and she tried, but clearly there was still some residual impairment as her smile was not normal.

They checked her sight. She had lost sight in her left eye the previous evening, but during this assessment, she had already re-gained some sight in the left eye. This was a simple test: with one eye covered, Alicia reported when she could see a finger moving left and right.

Dr. Rivera asked her to talk, and she began to talk in short sentences. She could not do any of these things the previous evening. Again, I got a big lump in my throat and began to tear up. I simply broke down in tears because the dramatic change was so impressive. We had thought the previous evening Alicia might end up permanently paralyzed for the rest of her life. But, here we were twelve hours later, and she was doing many things she could not do the previous evening. You could tell that she was not totally out of the anesthesia and that she would likely show further improvement later in the day. I believe the initial stroke assessment score was ten or eleven (out of 42).

As the anesthesia wore off, she did continue to improve. It was like watching someone wake up from anesthesia. It was not like she had amnesia. She had her knowledge. She just had to work harder to pull thoughts together and then deliver them via speech.

One thing that causes a problem when you have so many people who love you: they care about you and want to support you when you have something bad happen. Alicia has hundreds of friends and many close friends – from many years raising children, from the equestrian community and others she has known since childhood. I have said a number of times that "Everyone loves Alicia."

Alicia's children came by Wednesday. Sandy visited for a while and then left her to get some rest. Since her son Grant was local, he came by later when he got off work. They were glad to see their mom was recovering so well. Grant was particularly impressed since he had seen his mother in Northside Hospital ER during the onset of the stroke when she was partially paralyzed.

Dr. Nogueira came by to see Alicia around noon. I told Alicia that Dr. Nogueira had done the procedure to remove the clot, and she thanked him. He showed her the photos on his iPhone that he took during the procedure (and included earlier in this book), and she said, "Those are the clots that were in my brain?" She could not believe it. I thanked Dr. Nogueira again for all he did to save Alicia's life.

A couple of Alicia's friends came by on Wednesday and Thursday including Eleanor Effinger, Mary Portman, Susan Traynor and Linda Keefe. A number of her other friends all wanted to come visit, but I could tell that Alicia was weak from the ordeal. It would have been too stressful to Alicia to see so people coming by all the time so I asked a number of them to wait a few days so she could gain some strength.

During Eleanor's visit, Alicia said to her, "Can you believe I had to have a stroke to get my family together?" They both laughed over it. Eleanor thought that Alicia demonstrating humor was a good sign.

Alicia spent a lot of time sleeping. After all, the clot lodged in the base of her brain had caused tremendous stress on her entire brain, which in turn, triggered stress throughout her body. There was a small guest room as part of the ICU where I could go and sit while she was sleeping. I spent that time talking to friends and family as well as trying to get caught up on email. I remember taking a lunch break in mid-afternoon and going to the Grady cafeteria. I realized I had not eaten much in the past 24 hours. Somehow, I have managed to remember exactly what I had to eat that day: some salad, a baked potato and half a sandwich. The meal was not elegant, but it tasted really good.

When Alicia would awaken from resting, I gave her an update on the people I had talked with while she was sleeping. One humorous thing that Alicia mentioned was that if they let her go home on Friday, we could drive to DeBordieu Club in Georgetown, South Carolina and make it to the Blythe Wedding. My first reaction was to think, "Are you crazy? You can't have brain surgery on Tuesday night and expect to go to a wedding in South Carolina on Friday. That's a six hour drive!"

Connie and Frank Blythe live in Charlotte, and their son was getting married on Saturday evening. It's a good six to seven hour trip, and I could not imagine putting Alicia through that. She mentioned it a few times – it seemed to Alicia that it was her duty to do everything she could to be there for the wedding of her Blythe family wedding.

I told Alicia that it was unreasonable to drive that far after just getting out of the hospital. Plus, Hurricane Irene was expected on Friday to come through South Carolina and the Georgetown, SC area. Later, we found out from Connie that when the hurricane came through on Friday afternoon, they moved the rehearsal dinner from an outdoor tent to inside the club.

I stayed at the hospital until around 8:00 pm on Wednesday. Our pet sitter, Tamara Stewart, was kind enough to go by the house mid-day while Alicia was in the hospital to let Fritzie out and give her a walk so I did not have to drive back home from Grady.

I could really feel the effects of not getting enough sleep the previous night. Alicia was already asleep, so I left and got some dinner on the way home. When I got in bed, Angel came up, looked for her mommy and then proceeded to come over and knead on Alicia's pillow, just as she had done the previous night. She loved and missed Alicia.

On Thursday, Dr. Randy Martin came by to see Alicia. They talked a bit about their children going to Westminster and how Randy and I had worked together at the Cooper Clinic in Dallas years earlier. It was amazing that both Alicia and I had known Randy for many years before Alicia and I got back together.

He told Alicia that he wanted to do some tests starting this week to see if he could determine what caused the clot to form in the first place. He felt the stroke was most likely caused was by atrial fibrillation.

The attending Neurologist, Dr. Lisa Rivera, came by to do another stroke assessment. The score was less – around five or six. She talked to Alicia and me about her stroke and, in particular, her recovery. She wanted Alicia to know that she was extremely lucky to be sitting up in bed with the return of most neurologic and muscular function just a day after having the stroke and the procedure to remove the clot that caused it.

Alicia kept asking one question over and over again, "Why did this happen to me?" That is the subject of the next chapter.

Chapter 6

"WHY DID THIS HAPPEN TO ME?"

"Just give me a reason
Just a little bit's enough"

PINK with Nate Ruess, *Just Give Me a Reason*
Reprinted by permission.

We received some great news on Thursday afternoon, August 25, 2011: Dr. Rivera and the Neurology Team felt that Alicia's condition had improved enough that she was moved from the ICU to a standard post-stroke recovery room. The scene is shown in Figure 6-1. Upon first glance, it would appear that is a major problem and four medical staff members are working on her. But, if you look closely, you can see that they are simply sliding her from the ICU bed to the standard room bed. The nurse in the front is holding the IV equipment.

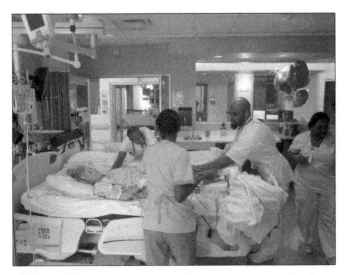

Figure 6-1. ICU staff moving Alicia from ICU to standard room on Thursday, Aug. 25, 2011. Alicia's stroke score had improved enough that she did not need ICU services any longer.

When we got settled into the standard post-stroke recovery room, Alicia started to reflect on the ordeal. She kept saying, "Why in the world did this happen to me?" It's a natural reaction to wonder what caused the stroke. She knew it had been serious, but her concern was more a reflection on the fact that she was living a positive, healthy lifestyle which would seem to prevent something like a stroke from ever happening to her.

"I eat right, don't smoke, exercise regularly, have kept my weight about the same as I was in high school, have low cholesterol levels and don't have much anxiety. Why would someone with a life profile like mine end up having a stroke?"

That question became the central theme of the post-stroke recovery. Everyone wanted to know what caused the stroke. Now, a couple of years after the stroke, we have pretty good idea what caused the stroke, but we cannot prove it.

Dr. Frankel and attending resident Dr. Lisa Rivera discussed this issue just about every time they came to check up on her. They told her that some people have very low risk factors and lived an active, healthy life but still suffer a stroke. They kept telling Alicia that the stroke was not likely due to her life style and risk factors but from some other reason.

When Dr. Frankel asked her if she suffered headaches or migraine headaches in the past, Alicia did have bouts of migraines in years past but mostly much earlier in life, not in the few years preceding the stroke. She told Dr. Frankel that she had headaches all the time and had to take an Excedrin most every day. Her comment was true strategically but not tactically. This was a good example of Alicia being able to communicate after the brain surgery but unable to get the facts correct in detail.

She was right about having had migraines and taking Excedrin. She always kept them in the car and on the nightstand, but the frequency of the migraines had fallen off since we had gotten together in 2006. I had to give Dr. Frankel an edited version of Alicia's comments.

Alicia had a few more visitors on Thursday afternoon and on Friday. Alicia's brother came by to pay a visit. He had been at Northside Hospital, and he was amazed to see his sister recovering so fast from a major stroke. Bruce always had such a positive attitude. Everyone is smiling when he is around. He often comes into a room and says, "Hey, hey, hey," while smiling, as in "OK everyone, the party can begin – I'm here now." Bruce always has a story or two to share and one of his favorite things is to play games – not football or basketball or board games but scavenger hunt games. He sometimes got his kids and grandkids scouting all over Atlanta to find something in order to get another clue.

Bruce had been a Georgia Tech fan since the days that his dad took him to Tech football games before there were any professional sport teams in Atlanta. Bruce started college at the University of Florida on a golf scholarship, but moved to the University of Georgia where he graduated. That, naturally, brought up the conundrum that he is now a Georgia graduate and expected to become a Georgia fan. Georgia graduates do not support Georgia Tech. It is just not done.

Well, here we are more than forty years after graduating from Georgia, and Bruce still has season tickets to Georgia Tech. He is such a dedicated fan that he has his own Yellow Jacket outfit. When he puts on the outfit, he looks like a gigantic Yellow Jacket. Families often take photos of him with their kids. Every year, Alicia and Bruce talked about how their favorite team was going to win in the annual Tech-Georgia football game. They make their traditional one dollar bet every year.

Bruce spent time with Alicia while she was recovering in the hospital talking about his youth, being the Georgia amateur champion in golf and playing in the high school national championship. We often wished that Bruce could have turned pro because we believe that his skill combined with this positive attitude would have led to his success on the pro tour.

I am sure Bruce was disturbed seeing his sister in a post-stroke condition, but he did not let on. What I think meant the most to both Bruce and me was that Alicia was able to talk about her past growing up which let Bruce know that her basic memory and personality were all there. Being able to practice using her brain to recall old memories helped her gain confidence that she was going to recover eventually from this serious medical incident.

Alicia's friend Bonnie Kerr Zarate came to visit and brought a cute little gift of a plastic box of jellybeans with a small teddy bear. Bonnie worked in the barn where Alicia rode her horse for a number of years and has remained a friend. The funny thing about her gift was that we typically don't eat jellybeans so the gift stayed in a cabinet at our house until we moved. We joked about the gift being the longest lasting one she got from someone following her stroke.

I stayed at Grady all day while Alicia was in the hospital. Our dog sitter, Tamara Stewart, assisted by coming by the house mid-day and taking Fritzie for a walk. I would take a break and go down to the Grady Cafeteria to get something to eat. I brought my laptop computer and iPhone to the hospital in order to stay up on important business issues and still be there for Alicia. Alicia's daughter Sandy came by as well to visit and give her mom support.

By Friday afternoon, Alicia's spirits began to improve. She reflected on her situation and began to appreciate the level of medical care she was receiving.

We have both laughed quite a bit when we look at the photo (Figure 6-2.) since she was in the hospital. She often says, "I looked horrible. Someone looking at it would think I've had a stroke!"

Alicia was starting to eat normally, but I could tell she was still in "recovery from trauma" mode. She was a bit slow in her responses and

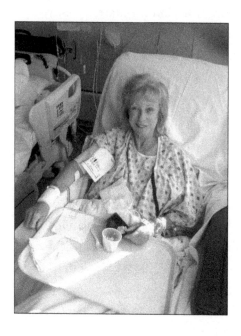

Figure 6-2. Friday, Aug. 26, 2011. Alicia's spirits are improving. She's trying to smile because she's just been told she could go home on Saturday, Aug. 27. There is still some impairment in facial muscle control which we found out later would return to normal within a few weeks.

while talking in her beautiful southern accent, her commentary seemed to drift around the subject.

Dr. Frankel had called Dr. Randy Martin to discuss her case. They decided to do a Trans-Esophageal Echocardiography (TEE) on Friday, August 26, 2011. The TEE test would allow the doctors to see if there were any other clots still in Alicia's heart that would possibly cause another stroke in the near-term. They also wanted to see if the TEE would show any signs of what originally had caused the stroke.

Because the clot lodged in the right Medial Cerebral Artery (MCA), it most likely was created in her heart, broke loose and traveled up from the heart through the right carotid artery into the MCA and then became lodged in the base of the brain in a smaller artery.

The TEE is one of main tests used in patients with unexplained stroke to see if the clot or other abnormalities inside the heart caused the stroke. TEE produces amazing results because it puts the echo transceiver down the esophagus and rests directly behind the heart. When you do a traditional echocardiogram from outside the chest, the ribs and lungs get in the way thus obscuring the image.

Dr. Martin is one of the pioneers of the TEE procedure. He currently is affiliated with Piedmont Heart Institute and is Past President of the American Society of Echocardiography. He was Professor of Medicine in Cardiology for twenty years at Emory Medical School. He felt that doing the TEE would either help identify what had caused the stroke or help rule out the possibility that additional clots were present in Alicia's heart that could suddenly cause an additional stroke.

As I mentioned earlier, it is rather ironic that both Alicia and I knew Randy before Alicia and I got back together at our forty fifth high school reunion in 2006. I worked with Randy from 1973-1975 at the Cooper Clinic in Dallas. Randy was an aspiring young physician doing exercise stress tests there. I had just finished my Ph.D. at Stanford. Since Randy was interested in doing a Cardiology Fellowship, I introduced him to

Dr. Don Harrison who was head of Cardiology at Stanford Medical School. I was able to meet and interact with Dr. Harrison when I was working with an organization that was setting up preventive medicine centers around the country.

Randy went to Stanford, became board certified in Cardiology and specialized in non-invasive technologies. He spent time at the University of West Virginia to set up a non-invasive cardiology lab and practice and then did similar work at the Mayo Clinic before settling down in Atlanta and spending more than twenty years working and teaching at Emory Medical School.

Alicia's knew Randy's daughter through Westminster. Alicia interacted with both Randy and his wife Ann. Thus, both Alicia and I had interacted with Randy and his family independently.

The Grady Cardiology Department conducted the TEE procedure on Friday morning, Aug. 26. Dr. Dimitri Cassimatis, Assistant Professor of Cardiology at Grady (and Emory), led the team that included observation by a number of Emory Medical School students.

It is difficult to watch the TEE procedure for the first time, although the procedure is not painful. The first thing they did was to anesthetize Alicia's throat. They had Alicia swallow a strong anesthetic. After a short time, the mouth, throat and esophagus become numb. The TEE team then inserted a small probe into the mouth and had Alicia swallow it. Although Alicia could not feel any pain, she could feel the uncomfortable pressure of the probe.

Once the probe passed the trachea, the TEE team let it descend down toward the stomach – the same way food travels down the esophagus. The TEE team then turned on the echo probe so they could record an echocardiograph that looked directly into Alicia's heart from the esophagus.

Honestly, I had to look away a number of times. Alicia was a real champ throughout the entire time which totaled thirty to forty minutes.

After the probe was placed directly behind the heart, Dr. Cassimatis and his team were able to look directly into Alicia's heart's chambers and get a high resolution view of the walls and the motion of the heart's beating muscles. Once the TEE team got the recordings they needed, they simply pulled the probe out.

Dr. Frankel came by to review the results of all the tests. He felt that the cause of the clot could not be determined. However, the TEE test did not find any further clots in Alicia's heart. The clot could have been formed in a random episode of atrial fibrillation where the upper chambers of the heart, the atria, beat at a very rapid, chaotic rate potentially leading to clot formation inside the left atrium. Or, it

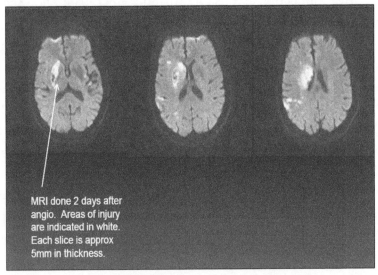

MRI done 2 days after angio. Areas of injury are indicated in white. Each slice is approx 5mm in thickness.

Figure 6-3. Friday afternoon, Aug. 26, 2011. MRI taken of Alicia's brain. The three images represent a slice approximately 5mm thick. The white area in each slice is the area damaged by the stroke. The clot stopped blood circulation that, in turn, killed neurons in the area, which cannot be recovered. The white area is cloudy and not solid so Alicia's brain has the ability to find new pathways through this area over time.

could have been biochemical. As Dr. Frankel said, "We know something caused a clot to form. We're just not exactly sure what it was."

On Friday afternoon, the medical team did another MRI and CT scan. They wanted to verify that the damaged area due to the stroke had not changed. This MRI was required in order to approve Alicia's discharge.

The neurology team, led by Dr. Lisa Rivera, did another stroke assessment late Friday afternoon and pronounced that she was doing so well that she would be allowed to go home on Saturday.

Consequentially, emotions swelled up and poured out from everything that had happened over the past three days. I started crying uncontrollably. Dr. Rivera told me it was perfectly normal to have such strong feelings, especially since Alicia had suffered a stroke just three days earlier and was now in a good enough condition that she could be discharged and return home. Dr. Rivera reviewed the medications she was prescribing for Alicia to take when home. She started Alicia on two medications: Simvastatin and Citalopram plus one aspirin.

She explained that there were a number of studies done on stroke survivors. Simvastatin – a statin normally used to lower blood lipids in people with high cholesterol – helps build the vitality of the arteries in the brain after a stroke. Citalopram, an antidepressant, has been shown to enhance neurovascular regeneration and sensory motor function after an ischemic stroke (a stroke caused by a clot vs. a stroke caused by a rupture in an artery in the brain). It enhances neurogenesis, neural cell migration and neurovascular repair. Both medicines would be taken long-term along with the single aspirin which acts to prevent the formation of clots. Dr. Rivera and Dr. Frankel recommended that Alicia stop taking her hormone replacement therapy (HRT) as that could have been a risk factor for causing a stroke.

On Saturday, Aug. 27, Alicia was approved to be discharged. The nursing team completed the discharge forms, and Alicia's daughter

Sandy helped her mom get dressed. I was able to take a photo of her son-in-law Grant and daughter Sandy with the nursing team. The photo is shown in Figure 6-4.

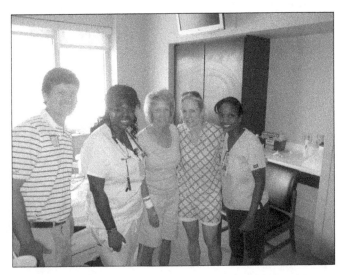

Figure 6-4. Saturday, Aug. 27, 2011 at 2:21 pm. Alicia is dressed and ready to leave Grady Hospital and the Marcus Stroke Center. Son-in-law Grant pictured on left with one nurse, Alicia, her daughter Sandy and another Grady nurse. While Alicia looks as if she isn't so happy, she was actually very happy to go home. Her face still shows signs of the effect of the stroke.

Dr. Michael Frankel told us to put Alicia's recovery in perspective, "Patients don't typically leave here in four days. Four weeks maybe but not four days. You all don't have the perspective I do. I see all of our stroke victims and very few of them have the recovery that you have experienced. We hope to have more of them going forward once the stent retriever clot removal device is formally approved. It's because of your high state of health that you were able to respond to the procedure in such a positive way that you're leaving here today."

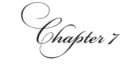

Chapter 7

RETURNING HOME

"And all along I believed I would find you
Time has brought your heart to me
I have loved you for a thousand years
I'll love you for a thousand more"

Christina Perri & David Hodges, *A Thousand Years*
Reprinted by permission.

Leaving Grady

I remember driving back to Grady Hospital on Saturday morning, August 27, 2011 and feeling how lucky we were to be taking Alicia home four days after the onset of her stroke. When I looked up at the massive hospital complex, I realized that there were many stroke victims lying in beds on the eighth floor that had been there for weeks and many would remain there for many more weeks. But, here we were with Alicia, leaving the Marcus Stroke Center only four days after she had been admitted.

Sure, four days in a hospital is quite typical for a most surgical procedures, but we were lucky to be able to have Alicia return home so quickly.

I asked Dr. Frankel about Alicia's prognosis. She clearly looked like she has been through a lot and while well enough perhaps to go home, she clearly was not fully recovered from the stroke.

Dr. Frankel told Alicia, "You should make a full recovery. But, realize that it's going to take many months. There will be a lot of physical improvement over the coming weeks – including getting your smile to return to normal, developing fine motor skills, but you're also going to find significant mental improvements for a year or even two after the stroke."

I was dumbfounded by his comment that we would notice changes a year or two later. Whenever I have had a surgical procedure such as my right knee being repaired for a torn meniscus, it hurt for a while but I fully recovered in a few weeks. This was ten times as long.

I have to say that I thought Dr. Frankel's saying we would see real improvement a year or more later was just some comforting statement – perhaps for a few small things. Well, as I'm writing this book more than two years after her stroke, Alicia just said something that she has not said once since she had her stroke.

Alicia has always been very organized. She loves to make lists of things to do, places to go and friends to meet. Everyone who has known Alicia for a long time knows that she is always on top of everything.

One of her pet phrases is, "We have to get organized!" to which she would immediately start planning her next painting, party or our move to our winter home in Wellington, FL. Her "We have to get organized!" phrase is a true statement of multi-tasking. It is where her brain is making simultaneous demands on different areas of the brain at the same time in order to what needs to happen to put on that dinner party or make sure everything is identified that we need for our relocation to Florida (or the reverse when we return to our home in Atlanta).

Dr. Frankel told both of us that multi-tasking is the last thing that returns in stroke recovery because it requires reestablishing connections from lots of different areas of the brain. It begins with just being able to make a short list of what to buy at the grocery store and gets much more complex such as the projects Alicia loved to organize for many years.

We were driving back to our home in Smyrna in early November 2012 – fully fifteen months after the stroke – when Alicia all of a sudden realized that we had Thanksgiving happening in a few weeks, relocation to south Florida in mid-December and the Christmas season upon us with ads already starting for "Black Friday" shopping. She turned to me and said, "We really have to get organized. There is so much to do over the coming weeks."

I smiled and said, "I don't believe it."

She responded, "You don't believe what?"

I replied, "I'm really very surprised to hear you say, 'We have to get organized' all on your own. Do you realize that you haven't said that phrase since before the stroke and that you have now used it for the first time since your stroke?"

Her saying an important phrase like that demonstrated that what Dr. Frankel said was correct: it does take many months – in this case over a year – for multi-tasking to begin to return in full form. So, if you have a family member who has had a stroke, and the doctors give a positive prognosis, then you need to realize that recovery is a very long process – perhaps lasting years. It is very affirming to see real improvements come about after a long time. It reinforces the fact that recovery is continuing.

On the other side, do not kid yourself into believing that the stroke-affected person is going to return to being exactly the same person as before the stroke. In Alicia's case, she has returned to what anyone would call "normal," but even in her very lucky outcome, she's a "new normal'" where some things are perfectly OK, but those normal things are composed of a few personality traits different than before. In Alicia's case, she is totally aware of these changes, e.g. "You know, I'm not as intense as I was before."

This change was perfectly normal, but it's a bit different than the way she was before the stroke. Before, she was always what I would consider an intense person. She would say things definitively. If you did not do something she wanted done, she would remind you about it over and over again until it was done. The intensity never caused an augment, but it was a noticeable trait.

Now, after the stroke, Alicia is less intense, but in a good way. She is more mild mannered. We both have said that this small change is a positive outcome from the stroke. It is a small thing: no one else would really notice it. Alicia is just as wonderful a person as ever. But, it is a good example of the small, but definitive changes that have happened as a result of the stroke.

Both Alicia and I were impressed with the flood of help and assistance. There are some details about the assistance we received in Chapter 8 – Becoming Overwhelmed, but I know I cried with appreciation when friends would take their own time to come visit, bring some food or simply help us out for a short time. While you may need to control the level of assistance, realize that your friends (and some who may only be acquaintances) will reach out so accept their gifts graciously.

Arriving Home

We arrived home around mid-day on Saturday, August 27, 2011. We had a number of family and friends there to help Alicia get settled in. You can see the scene in Figure 7-1. Kathy Sands was there to visit with her. Kathy has been a good friend for over thirty years. You can see Alicia looks tired in the picture. But also notice that a number of family and friends are in the background. They brought food, love and friendship. Even our dog Fritzie wanted to be part of the welcoming committee.

Alicia's daughter Sandy and her husband Grant came to the hospital to assist her in getting ready to leave. They also were there to help her get comfortable at home. Alicia's brother came by as well. He had a number of stories and jokes to share, and Linda Keefe, who was at the Marcus Stroke Center with Alicia's son Grant and me, came by with some food.

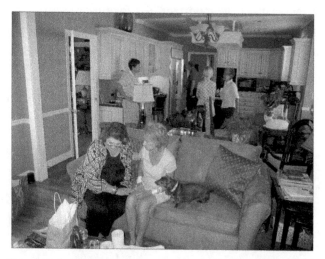

Figure 7-1. Scene right after coming home from the hospital. Kathy Sandsvisiting with Alicia with Fritzie. In the background are Alicia's son-in-law Grant, Brother Bruce Grant, daughter Sandy and Linda Keefe are shown in the kitchen.

Now, take a look at Figure 7-2. It shows Alicia taking a nap on the family room sofa. This became her main location for most of the day for many weeks following her returning home from Grady Hospital. While we all love and cherish taking a nap in the afternoon every once and a while, Alicia was taking three or four hour-long naps a day.

Dr. Frankel pointed out that the body uses naps to help the brain recover from the stroke. It makes sense. Since Alicia's brain was damaged, sleep was one of her most important tools to get well. During the nap, the brain would "wash out" some of the damaged area by rerouting connections as well as helping putting new neurons to work by connecting them up in ways to work around the compromised area.

I would sometimes see Alicia get up from a nap, take a walk with the dogs, return to the house and take another nap. I always encouraged Alicia to take naps. It is important in stroke recovery to refrain from saying things like, "You nap all the time." Rather, you should encourage as many naps as possible as it helps the brain deal with the trauma and begin to recover.

After many weeks, the frequency of the naps fell off from perhaps three or four a day down to one or two. Alicia still takes a nap in the

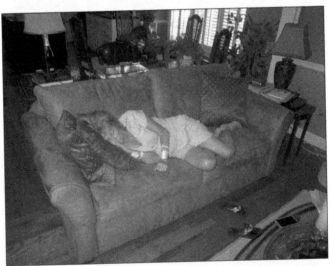

Figure 7-2. Saturday afternoon, Aug. 27 - Alicia taking a nap after returning from the hospital. Sometimes Alicia would take three or four naps a day. Naps were an important as a way for the brain to recover from the trauma of a stroke.

afternoon most every day after she rides her horse, part for physical recuperation and partly for brain recovery as well.

We decided to eat dinner outdoors on Saturday, Aug. 27, 2011. It was a nice end of summer day in Atlanta as it had cooled off just a bit but was still pleasant. Since Grant and Sandy were there, I had one of the kids take a photo of Alicia and me as shown in Figure 7-3.

This photo clearly shows the post-stroke effect on facial muscles. The stroke was on the right side of her brain which affected the movement on the left side of her body. And, one of the most prominent places which this is noticeable is in the face. In this photo, which has become the "poster child" photo that shows the damage to Alicia's body, Alicia is trying to smile. She has full control over her right side, so she's lifted her cheek muscles. But, being compromised on the left side, the smile is sagging a bit as well as bulging due to lack of small muscle control.

Alicia was not in any pain and in overall in good spirits (other than being tired and taking naps). Alicia remembers this as a positive, enjoyable experience for her since she was surrounded by family and friends. In other words, her image of the situation did not align with the physical appearance to others. She looks at this photo and says, "Geez, it looks like I had a stroke." It is both comical but also perceptive that her image internally of herself was relatively normal, while others were obviously looking at someone who was compromised, different from the Alicia they knew before the stroke. The good news is that Alicia regained her normal smile within a few weeks mostly due to practicing to "over smile" in which got her left side facial muscles to respond. You'll notice the difference in the later photographs.

There are a couple of interesting things to notice in Figure 7-4. While this is simply another picture taken on Saturday, Aug. 27 during dinner, it shows a casserole dish that was brought by the house so Alicia (and I) would not have to cook or go out. Also, you can see that both Grant and Sandy are smiling in a way that looks natural and not forced.

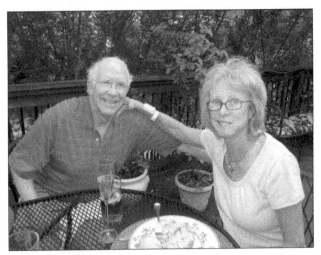

Figure 7-3. Saturday evening, Aug. 27 - Having dinner after leaving Grady Hospital. This has become Alicia's classic "post-stroke" photo. Alicia was very happy to be home. Note that while her face looks deformed on the right side, it is the left side that was compromised and unable to move the same way as her right side.

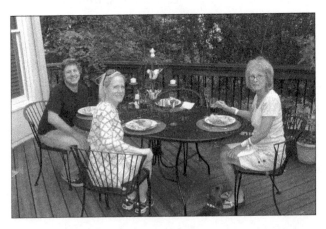

Figure 7-4. Saturday evening, Aug. 27 - Alicia with her son Grant and daughter Sandy. Our Dachshund Fritzie was begging as usual. The weather was typical late August inAtlanta – hot in the day and warm in the evening.

They were truly happy that their mother was doing all right. They are relaxed and not stressed. Their attitude helped Alicia to recover faster. She was accepted by her family and friends. I reminded her over and over again that her facial muscles would return to normal in a matter of weeks to a few months. And, of course, you can see our dog Fritzie is looking for a handout from Alicia. This photo was taken on the same porch where Alicia suffered her stroke.

Figure 7-5 shows Alicia going back to bed after breakfast to lie down in the bed rather than to take a nap on the family room sofa. Also note that our white cat Angel did her part to help Alicia recover. She sat on the pillow next to Alicia's head almost every time she took a nap in the bed. Angel stayed on Alicia's pillow most nights as if she knew her "mommy" was hurting and recovering.

Cats have a sense of interpreting the situation in almost a surreal manner. No one ever asked or told Angel to sleep on Alicia's head but she did it all the time. She still sleeps on Alicia's pillow for part of every

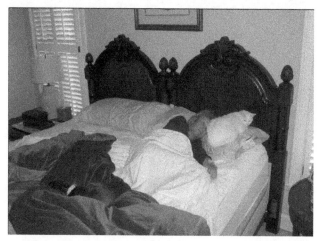

Figure 7-5. Sunday morning, Aug. 28, 2011 – the day after coming home from the hospital. Note how our cat Angel was so glad to have her "mommy" home. She sat there on Alicia's pillow day and night to help her recover.

night. In fact, almost every night when we get ready to go to bed, Angel jumps up on the bed and makes her "grand entrance" coming over to sit on Alicia's pillow or move over to the bed stand where she drinks out of a glass we put there. She has a habit of drinking out of this glass as part of her evening ritual which we call "Angel drinking her 'kitty water.'" We laugh about it because her little cat metal name tag hangs from her collar and jingles from hitting the edge of the glass.

Remember, if someone in your family is home recovering from stroke, he or she may go back to bed for naps soon after getting up. Nothing is wrong, and they are not likely having another stroke (unless he or she shows definitive signs of another stroke occurring). Naps are normal and will become less frequent over time.

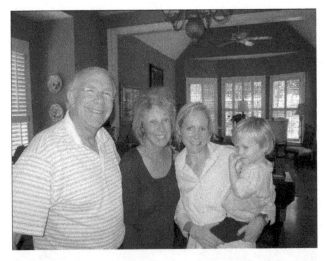

Figure 7-6. Sunday afternoon, Aug. 28 – the day after coming home from the hospital. The author with Alicia, her daughter Sandy and her son Grant. We had started an exercise for Alicia to "over smile" to practice flexing her facial muscles. While this looks a bit stroke-like, this turned out to help Alicia get her smile back to normal. Still, it took a number of months to completely recover.

Figure 7-6 shows Alicia next to Sandy and her son Grant the day after she came home from the hospital (Sunday, Aug. 28, 2011). Alicia is trying to smile. I had reminded her to try hard to smile, and you can see that she's "over smiling" in the photo. What she did was over smile on her right side in which she had full control of her facial muscles but the left side "lagged behind" causing her to look more unnatural than if she had not tried to smile at all. But, these exercises really helped Alicia to think about moving her left facial muscles. Sometimes, Alicia would stand in front of a mirror and try to smile over and over again as an exercise to get the left side muscles working again. This exercise helped her smile to return to normal.

Figure 7-7 shows a number of friends (but certainly not all) who came by to visit with Alicia after she returned home from the hospital. What is interesting in these photos is the range of fine facial muscle

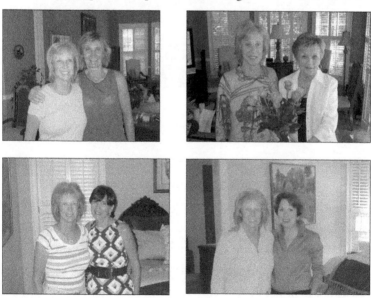

Figure 7-7. Alicia with friends (clockwise) Nina Macrae, Lorellee Wolters, Lynn Ford and Susan Traynor. Note that Alicia's smile is sometimes noticeably off & sometimes almost back to normal.

control Alicia demonstrated. Some look very "stroke like" while others are much more normal.

Figure 7-8 shows Alicia smiling about two weeks after the stroke. Clearly there are signs that she is regaining more control over her facial muscles. This has become the one photo that shows real improvement from the others in Alicia's ability to smile.

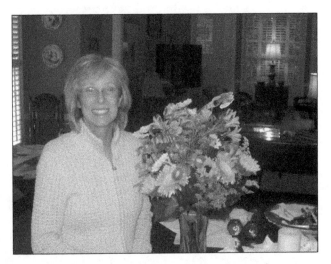

Figure 7-8. Flowers from Bryan and Claudia Purdy on Sept. 7. Over smiling a bit but showing more facial control.

On September 10, I decided that Alicia should have a day at the hair dresser and go out to dinner. Immediately after the stroke, Alicia did not spend much time with personal grooming. She was napping all the time. You could see positive, although small, changes after most of her naps.

Alicia set up an appointment with Michael Azar, hair stylist extraordinaire in Atlanta who she has known for many years. She really looked great that evening when we went to have dinner at our favorite restaurant, Houston's Paces Ferry. While there was still a little lag in her left facial muscles (Figure 7-9), you can see a much more relaxed person than she had been since the stroke and someone who enjoys how she looks.

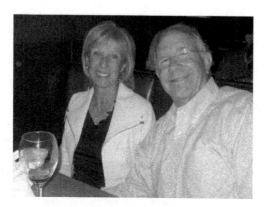

Figure 7-9. Taking Alicia out to our favorite restaurant, Houston's after she got her hair done at Michael's on Saturday, Sept. 10, two weeks after returning home. You can clearly see improvement in facial muscle control.

By September 15, 2011 Alicia did not need to consciously work on smiling. Her ability to smile was now very close to being back to normal. You can see this in Figure 7-10. Alicia went out to lunch with Eleanor Effinger. They went to Nancy G's, one of our favorite local restaurants.

Eleanor, along with Kathy Sands, had stayed up all night on Aug. 23, 2011 calling me every hour to get an update on Alicia's progress at the Marcus Stroke Center. You can see Alicia is happy and not over smiling any longer.

By the end of September, Alicia was conducting her daily life more like she was before the stroke. She still did not have multi-tasking back, but she was feeling better and taking fewer naps.

The one problem that I did not expect became a huge issue for me: how to deal with Alicia's recovery and still do the things that I normally did before she had the stroke. The next chapter discusses my becoming overwhelmed from all the responsibilities for caring for Alicia while trying to do everything I was doing before the stroke.

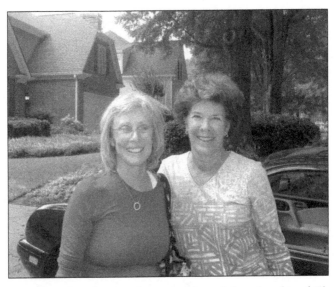

Figure 7-10. Alicia being taken to lunch with her close friend Eleanor Effinger around Sept. 15. Eleanor was one of the friends who stayed up all night following the surgery, waiting to hear if it was successful.

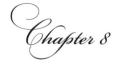

BECOMING OVERWHELMED

"I'm only a man in a silly red sheet
Digging for kryptonite on this one way street
Only a man in a funny red sheet
Looking for special things inside of me
Inside of me, inside of me."

Five for Fighting, *Superman (It's Not Easy)*
Reprinted by permission.

The day after we got home from the hospital (on Saturday, Aug. 27, 2011), I needed to go to the grocery store to pick up a few items and then go swim at LA Fitness. This, of course, would not be any problem under normal circumstances. After all, I would only be gone around ninety minutes – an hour to swim and thirty minutes to go to the store. But, I remember feeling very frightened and scared to leave Alicia at home. I kept thinking, "What if she has another stroke while I'm gone?"

It was a strange feeling because on my logical side, I knew that she was on the way to recovery and could nap and do just fine with my being gone for one and a half hours. But, emotionally, I felt a sense of panic. There was also the caretaker responsibility: "What if she needed me while I was gone?" She was taking three or four naps a day at this point so there were not many requests for things I needed to do for her, but I felt a sense of guilt, of abandonment, like what you would feel if you left a small child at home alone.

The way I dealt with leaving home initially was to do things small tasks in a mad rush. Instead of going to work out and then going to the store, I would go swim and come immediately home and then take Alicia with me to the store. When I left to go swim, I put Alicia's iPhone phone right next to the sofa where she was napping so she could easily find it and send me a text message if she needed me for some reason.

Surprisingly, Alicia looked to be back to normal – other than when she smiled. She had all of her memory. Her long-term memory was completely intact.

At first, she did not have very much recall about when the stroke happened. She reflected on the day she had the stroke, "I went to sit on the back porch and remembered that I couldn't get up. I couldn't figure out how to get up. I'd say, 'OK, 1-2-3' and strain to get up, but nothing would happen. Details after that became fuzzy." As a result, I did not know how much damage resulted in Alicia's brain from the stroke. I had to be cautious.

I remember trying to sort through what was damaged and what was not affected. I thought to myself, "What was just part of being home right after surgery (any surgery)? and "When did she need help and when did she not need assistance?" I know that I was supposed to encourage her independence and not do too much for her, but I felt that helping her was a privilege because I loved her. There was a constant balancing act trying to encourage her to do things herself, e.g. "Why don't you see if you can set the table?" or "Can you remember which medications you are supposed to take?" and being a loving husband as in "Here, let me get that for you."

I thought to myself, "I love Alicia. I can take care of her, get all my work done and take time to work out and have some time for myself." I attacked the challenge with a vengeance. I felt I could manage this. After all, how hard could it be?

But after about a week of trying to be supportive, still get work done as well as workout and go run errands, I found it was simply "too much" to handle. I simply could not do it all. I realized at this point, "Whoa, this is taking more time and is far more difficult than I thought it would be to do everything."

You think you can do it all. You want to think you can do anything and everything. After all, you love the person, so you do not mind taking care of her, but I think most people in this situation finally realize that they simply cannot be a full-time caretaker and continue doing everything else that they had been doing in the past. I found I became overwhelmed with just the caretaking alone. It was easy to spend the entire day caring for her. But, you realize that you're also trying to run your own life. I had clients to contact, emails to answer, briefings with mobile and wireless vendors that fell further behind.

I have to say that I got to thinking, "This is more than I ever bargained for!" I can remember lying in bed at night staring at the ceiling and thinking, "How am I going to deal with all this?" It was building inside to the point of becoming overwhelming. At first, it was an exciting challenge, as in "Hey, I can take care of Alicia. It can't be that difficult to do. I am likely wasting time now and with a little focus, I will be able to check on her and continue doing everything that I did before."

I remember when I reached the point where I realized I could not both take care of Alicia and do what I was doing before. I did not have the ability to plan or consider what to do next. I felt I had stopped and become someone who could not get anything done.

I told Alicia that trying to do both was becoming very difficult for me and that, perhaps, we needed to get some part-time help to assist and make life easier for me and still provide the necessary care for her.

That is when Kathy Sands, one of Alicia's long-time friends, dropped by for a visit. She did not know it at the time, but she brought with her the solution to my problem. Kathy came with food she had made to help us out. Kathy is one of those wonderful friends who just does things for others, keeps smiling and does not ask for any credit. She is one of God's angels.

Enter Genna Brown

After she had put a ton of food down on the counter and a dinner in the refrigerator, she said something like, "I was at Wender & Roberts today, and there was a stack of cards on the counter from a gal looking for part-time work – caretaking, baby-sitting, going to the grocery store, etc." She handed me the card. The gal's name was Genna Brown. I told Kathy that it could be just what we needed.

I called Genna, and sure enough, she was available to help us out. She had been recently laid off at Wender & Roberts pharmacy where she had worked. I explained to her that I needed some part-time assistance with a number of things that were becoming overwhelming for me. At first, I felt a bit guilty for needing someone to help me, but if I were going to be able to take care of Alicia, do my work and take care of myself with an occasional workout, then I needed to let Genna help out.

Once she came to help, it was like a thousand pounds were lifted off my shoulders. I was still in the "worry wart" mode believing that something might happen to Alicia if I left her alone for thirty seconds. Part of that was from feeling guilty over not being at the house when

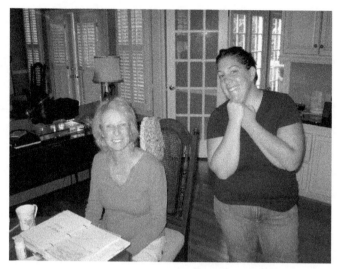

*Figure 8-1. Alicia with Genna Brown, our family
assistant who helped the author deal with being
overwhelmed and assisted Alicia with recovery exercises.*

she suffered the stroke. As it turned out, Alicia was not going to suffer another stroke, and it was perfectly all right for Genna and Alicia to spend time together without me playing the baby sitter.

One of the initial tasks was to help Alicia go through all of our mail order catalogs and throw out those we did not need (which was most of them). We had a ton of catalogs that had not been reviewed. Genna and I placed them in stacks in the family room, and Alicia would look at them when she did not feel too tired. She actually found a number of Christmas presents in them. They also served to give her an exercise to focus on as well as rid the house of clutter.

One of the things we were told at the Marcus Stroke Center at Grady Hospital was that planning and multi-tasking took the longest to be restored after a stroke since they are the most demanding on the cortex in the brain. I started asking Alicia to tell me what she was going to do a couple of times a day. I did not have her plan things out past the current day at first. Rather, I'd ask her, "What's happening today?" or "Do we have anything scheduled today?"

At first, Alicia's response was along the lines of, "I don't know," perhaps as a convenient way of not getting her brain to think about it. So, during the previous evening or in the morning I put something on the calendar for the next day, e.g. go to grocery store or out to dinner at Houston's. I would show it to her and then the next morning ask the same question, "What's scheduled for today?" If she was not sure, I would give her a hint. I would then ask her the same question a little later. I honestly think this helped, although we are now a few years past the stroke, and both Alicia and I know that her short-term memory is still a bit compromised.

Another thing we were told to do was to encourage Alicia to take a nap each day. We both found that rather humorous because Alicia almost always took a nap each afternoon after riding her horse. But, I really did not have to remind or encourage Alicia to take naps after she came home from the hospital. She became a "nap queen" taking as many as three or four a day.

Alicia would typically get up, get a cup of coffee and look at the paper. Then, she would go lie down and take a forty-five minute nap. She would wake up, do some things and then take another nap. She would take a nap after lunch and another nap late afternoon and still another after dinner before going to bed.

You could see that these naps were really helpful because she almost always woke up in a more conscious state: remembering more things, being more outgoing and laughing a lot.

One thing that Alicia did not do at all after the stroke was cry. She would express disappointment in her having a stroke but not fall into a crying fit. Alicia did not cry until the following March when we were in our Wellington, Florida home. She got a call from her mother's care taker, Shirley, telling her that her ninety-six-year old mother was not doing well and to please fly back to Atlanta. Alicia put down the phone and realized her mom was not going to be around much longer and began to cry.

Alicia's mother had been in failing health for some time. She had times when she was delirious saying that people with knives were coming to get her. I saw Alicia go through a rather slow, on-going grieving process, but when that call came requesting that she come back to Atlanta to say goodbye to her mom, she finally began to cry.

Alicia even noticed that it was the first time she had cried since the stroke, "Good grief, this is the first time I've cried since my stroke six months ago." Alicia flew back to Atlanta and met her mom with her brother Bruce. Her mom could only whisper, but Alicia told her mom that she loved her, and her mom whispered the same in response.

Alicia's mother (Jane Ebersole) held on until May 7, 2012 when she simply died in her sleep. After her mom passed away, Alicia did not go through a lot more grieving. She had grieved over her mom for the previous two months so when she finally passed away, it was more of a relief for her to not be in such a poor condition, unable to move or talk. Alicia was sad, of course, but there was not much more grieving to do.

Fixing Meals

One of the things that really helped with the post-stroke care was friends who pitched in to help fix meals. Alicia was and still is a five star cook in the family, and I am only good for fixing soup or a peanut butter sandwich.

But, Alicia's daughter Sandy came to the rescue by setting up meals through a handy web site called TakeThemAMeal.com. It's a non-profit site made to help people out with a short-term need. The site gets grants and donations. It is basically an online calendar in which friends of a family are sent an email inviting them to volunteer and bring a meal for a family or friend.

Figure 8-2 shows a screen shot from the web site: http://takethemameal.com/setup.php. Sandy set it up, and then we gave her some email addresses from friends who had offered to make a meal to help us out.

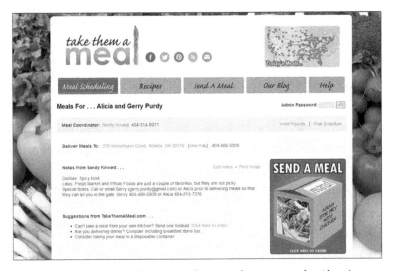

Figure 8-2. TakeThemAMeal.com web site set up by Alicia's daughter Sandy so friends could provide a meal.

Figure 8-3 shows the actual meal schedule from early September 2011 starting with Barbara Goldsmith, another of Alicia's long-term equestrian friends. Barbara lived in the house she grew up in on Nancy Creek Drive. Alicia used to live just around the corner on Ridgewood Road. Alicia would sometimes ride over to Barbara's house to use the riding ring. Barbara had a wonderful horse named Gretta. Remember that name. It comes up again in couple of chapters.

Barbara has a great recipe for spaghetti that she fixes in large volume and takes to the homeless shelter in Atlanta. She brought over a small sample of her normal batch. We had to laugh because it was enough to last two or three nights. We put the leftovers in the freezer and made two other dinners from it over the coming months. Honestly, everyone on the list brought a lot of food.

Date	Meal Provider		What I Plan To Bring (Or Send...)	Actions
Hide Previous Meals				
Mon, Aug 29	Barbara Goldsmith		Dinner	Change | Remove
Tue, Aug 30	Jill Harkey	770-605-2739	Chicken Divan, salad, rolls, and brownies	Change | Remove
Thu, Sep 1	mary portman	404-915-1443	fresh artichoke hearts, grilled chicken parmesan casserole and dessert	Change | Remove
Sat, Sep 3				Take | Send | Cancel
Mon, Sep 5				Take | Send | Cancel
Tue, Sep 6				Take | Send | Cancel
Thu, Sep 8	Susan Traynor	678-427-1580	Flank Steak Salad, rolls, fruit	Change | Remove
Sat, Sep 10	Nina Macrae	6787930695	Shepherds pie	Change | Remove
Mon, Sep 12	Mary Leslie Spencer	404-401-3373	herb baked chicken, bread, fruit, green beans	Change | Remove
Tue, Sep 13	Kristi Roche	404-931-3123		Change | Remove

Figure 8-3. Meal schedule in September 2011. What we found was that many meals lasted more than one day so that we adjusted the schedule to provide some free days to get caught up with the provided meals.

Short-Term Memory and Multi-Tasking

I found it helpful for Alicia to have and use a big calendar where she could see the entire month and write down major activities for each day in the month. As Alicia really got into using the calendar, started planning everything. It has served such a good function that we still use a large calendar today. It helps us to put the birthdays for all the kids, grandkids and spouses on the calendar at the start of the year so we do not forget them. We now have a total of something like thirty-one family member's birthdays on the calendar.

As I stated above, two issues seemed to take much longer to recover than all the others: 1) short-term memory and 2) multi-tasking. Of course, older people tend to forget things more than younger people so it is really hard at times to know whether Alicia forgot something owing to the stroke or getting older. I forget lots of things, but the difference is that after a stroke, it is hard to remember things that you just talked about versus the pervasive forgetting we all have where we put something down and cannot remember where.

But, a lapse in short-term memory can be somewhat dangerous. I had to take my first business trip in October (following Alicia's stroke on Aug. 23), and I hoped that nothing would go wrong. We had Genna Brown spend a little more time visiting during the day. But, that evening, Alicia accidently left a burner all night. While it did not cause any damage, it was still upsetting to have it happen. This was a case of simply forgetting to turn it off.

Whereas forgetting something on a short-term basis is typically not very serious, not being able to multi-task can be more serious: it is difficult to drive if you cannot multi-task since you have to do many things at the same time (although you get so used to it that you do not usually realize it). The next few chapters deal with a few good examples of the difficulty in dealing with multi-tasking, from rehab exercises to riding a horse to planning a social event.

I remember the time when Alicia drove home from the grocery store one Sunday afternoon. She appeared to handle it quite well, but I was quite stressed because I knew if there was something unusual like someone running a red light or someone who stopped suddenly in front of us, Alicia might not have the detailed motor-skills retrained to handle it.

Over the subsequent months, Alicia and I agreed to focus on short driving sessions that had little or no traffic. She slowly got more comfortable and began to drive places on her own.

Re-Engaging Socially

We also found it a bit challenging to go out with friends who knew Alicia had suffered a stroke. We did not want them to feel uncomfortable not knowing what to do or expect, so we focused on things that were with family and close friends. By Christmas 2011, Alicia had mostly returned to normal and going out or attending social events became more comfortable and similar to pre-stroke times.

We had one particularly enjoyable dinner on September 19, 2011 about a month after Alicia's stroke when we had dinner with Matt and Janet Burrell (Figure 8-4). You may recall from the night of the stroke that Matt is an oncology physician and was the doctor present in the emergency room who helped us deal with the situation. Going to dinner with them was pleasant because we really like both Janet and Matt, and we wanted to share with Matt everything that had happened after we left Northside Hospital for the Marcus Stroke Center on August 23.

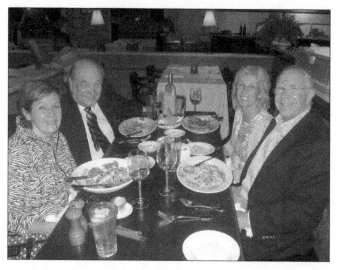

Figure 8-4. Dinner with Dr. Matt and Janet Burrell at Brio's in Atlanta on Sept. 19, 2011. Matt came to Northside Hospital on August 23 to help the family deal with the medical situation. He was the first to tell us to get Alicia to the Marcus Stroke Center at Grady Hospital after learning that radiology had found a clot in Alicia's Medial Carotid Artery (MCA).

Another pleasurable event was when Alicia's children took their mom out for brunch on her birthday at the Flying Biscuit restaurant on September 26, 2011 (Figure 8-5). You can see that Alicia has gotten her smile back to almost normal, and she really enjoyed getting together with her son Grant and her daughter Sandy.

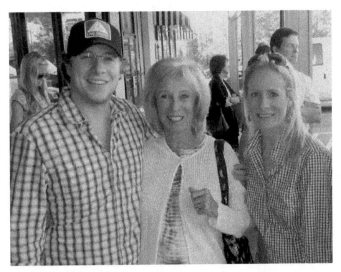

Figure 8-5. Alicia's birthday brunch on September 26, 2011 with son Grant and daughter Sandy at Flying Biscuit.

I think this get-together also helped reassure her children. They had not seen their mother since the stroke in August. They all talked with her a number of times, but this visit enabled them to see for themselves that she was recovering at a nice pace.

Alicia's rehabilitation process provides the next interesting path in her post-stroke recovery. That process is summarized in the next chapter.

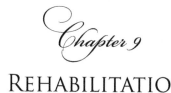

REHABILITATION

"Missed the Saturday dance
Heard they crowded the floor
Couldn't bear it without you
Don't get around much anymore"

Rod Stewart, *I Don't Get Around Much Anymore*
Reprinted by permission.

The orders when we left the Marcus Stroke Center at Grady Hospital were to begin rehabilitation. The specific rehab program was to be done via assessment and then treatment. Although there were a number of facilities that do post-stroke rehab, we decided to use the Rehabilitation Department at Northside Hospital since it was close to our home and had a good reputation.

It was a little strange walking back into Northside Hospital again since the entire process of dealing with and managing the stroke was at Northside Hospital just a week earlier. A full hospital rehab center deals

95

with recovering patients from a number of medical problems including heart attack, stroke and injury.

The initial session was focused on assessing Alicia's condition. She had assessment tests for walking up and down stairs, for fine motor skills, for control of her limbs and for mental and verbal capabilities.

I found the small pin test the most fascinating and one that clearly showed the damage to Alicia's control of her left side. There were little pins set in a wooden block. Each pin had a knob on the end of it that matched a cutout each hole in the wooden block. Each pin had to be picked up and then twisted with the two forefingers in order to get them into the holes. It seemed to me be a simple exercise.

Alicia started with her left hand. She picked up the pins and put them in the board by twisting her fingers so that the knob on the end of the pin would line up with the hole. The time it took to put the pins in the board was four minutes and twenty-five seconds. She then did the same exercise with her right hand. The time was strikingly different: one minute and fifteen seconds. It took Alicia almost three minutes longer to use her fine motor control with her left hand than with her right hand.

Alicia attended two sessions a week for about three weeks. After three weeks, the therapist repeated the assessments. The total time it took Alicia to complete the test using the pegs using her left hand gradually came down – from four to three to two minutes and, finally, to around one and a half minutes compared to one minute and fifteen seconds for the right hand.

Alicia's brain was going through a re-training exercise to request services around and through the area affected by the stroke. She consciously knew what to do but it took trying over and over to figure out how to get her fingers to work again doing such fine movements. I had to admit that it gave me a lump in my throat seeing the improvement from one week to the next. Figure 9-1 shows the occupational therapy nurse working with Alicia on cognitive activities like the small pin test.

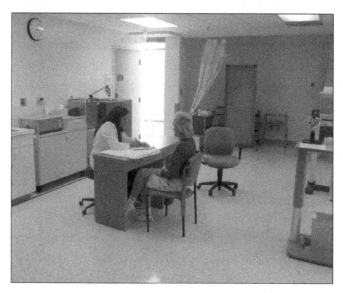

Figure 9-1. Alicia working in early September 2011 with the occupational therapy assistant following the stroke. Exercises were utilized to improve fine motor skills (see the one described in the text) and multi-tasking.

Alicia explained that she knew in her head what to do but she could not get the ends of her forefingers to cooperate and move as fast as she wanted them to. However, she could also notice the progress and was pleased to see that she was returning back to normal.

There is a big difference between learning something new versus retraining. In learning something knew, your brain does not know how to do something. Consequently, you have to build an awareness about it in your brain as well as practice doing it to get better at it. Retraining is different. When you're retraining as after a stroke, you already know how to do it. You previously could control the muscles to do it. You think in your head, "I know how to do this" but you cannot do it or do it nearly as well.

The network path from your brain to your muscles that had been previously set up has been interrupted. Retraining has the brain find a new pathway in order to get the muscles to do the same thing.

One of the best examples of this effort was Alicia trying to take out her soft contact lenses. She was able to put them in partly because all she needed to do was get the lens near the open eye, and the lens attached itself to the liquid in the eye.

However, when Alicia tried to take them out after having the stroke, she had a difficult time doing it. At first, I did the wrong thing by simply taking them out for her. I would clean off my fingers, hold her eye lid open and quickly touch the lower part of the eyeball, pinch the lens and pull it out, In order to get the lens out, I had to put my fingers close to but not actually touching the eye. I then drew my fingers across the outside of her eyeball and almost like magic the lens would stick to my dry fingers.

We did that for a while quite successfully, but I kept remembering the direction from the Marcus Stroke Center staff: do not do things for Alicia even though you can. Encourage her but let her do them herself.

Alicia clearly wanted to get back to being able to take out her contact lenses. I would let her try but sometimes, it would get frustrating. She would try and try but simply could not do it. I decided to watch her more closely when she was trying to take out her contact lenses. When I came up right beside her, I noticed that the thumb and first finger were too low compared to the center of her eye. She was pinching the lower eye lid area instead of the middle of her eye.

I asked her, "Where do you think you are putting your fingers to get out the contact lenses?"

She replied, "I'm putting them in the middle of my eye."

Clearly, she had problem with the fine motor control regarding taking out her contact lenses. Her brain thought she was placing her thumb and first finger in the middle of her eye, but, in fact, the fingers ended up at the bottom of her eye thus preventing her from successful pinching and successfully taking out her contact lens.

I took her fingers and placed them in the center of her eye with the upper eyelid raised to provide a clear path for the fingers to touch the contact lens. Bingo! She was able to pull out the lens on the first try. For the next few days, when she went to take out her contact lenses, I would remind her by saying, "Put your fingers in the middle of your eye." I would then re-position her fingers until they were, in fact, in the middle of her eye. After a few days of trying this, Alicia was able to put her fingers in the right place. It took some additional reinforcement, but she was able to re-learn this task and not need any further assistance from me. It appears that my repositioning her fingers resulted in feedback to her cortex telling her, "This is where you need to put your fingers, not where you thought you did before."

Another example: we decided to give our new Dachshund puppy Bella some puppy lessons. When the instructor told Alicia to hold her forearm at a right angle from her shoulder arm, she ended up with her forearm at more like one hundred thirty-five degrees or tilting down. Again, she thought that she was telling her forearm to be level.

I helped put her arm in the correct position level to the ground while walking Bella. It took about a few times before she was able to re-learn how to put the forearm in a level position, but once she picked it up, she did not need any further assistance with this task. Again, I believe that the adjustment in her forearm found an alternate pathway back to her cortex telling her where she needed to place her arm.

As previously noted, the physical therapy part of the rehab program initially included major physical movements like walking, climbing up and down steps, fine motor skills and speech therapy (Figure 9-2). It was surprising that Alicia made great progress in the gross motor skills area and recovered enough after about two or three weeks that she was told she didn't need any further physical therapy.

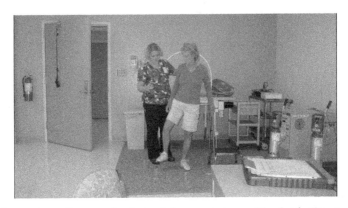

Figure 9-2. Alicia with physical therapy nurse at Northside Hospital. She was helping Alicia regain motor control and strength on her left side.

On the other hand, I wondered what the speech therapist was going to do because it seemed that Alicia did not have any problem talking after the stroke. Never the less, when we showed up to meet with her, I quickly found out that the therapy was more about cognitive skills than pure speech. The therapist did an interesting exercise where she showed Alicia a picture with a number of images. The therapist asked her to look at it for a minute. Then, she did some recognition skills where she was asked to find and explain what she saw in a series of images.

Overall, Alicia seemed to have good interpretive skills in place. Alicia was asked to recall the items she saw in the first image. The exercise was to test her short-term memory. At first she had problems remembering the items in the first image, but she got better over the following two weeks. Alicia did a number of exercises in both interpreting images and remembering things in the short term.

I recall that our good friend Eleanor Effinger brought over some children's learning books like <u>Finding Waldo</u> where Alicia had to find the Waldo figure in a collage of images and doing games like Concentration where Alicia had to remember where the picture after it had been revealed and then hidden again.

I would say that Alicia's one recurring problem is remembering recent things she hears - things that are stored and retrieved in the short-term memory. She could recall details of her growing up and most of the major events in her life with great detail but would have trouble remembering something that was said a few minutes earlier.

This kind of problem shows up when you put your keys down somewhere and then try to remember where you put them a few minutes later. To be sure, most of us have problems with remembering where we put something down much later, like many hours or the next day, but Alicia would have problems remembering things after just a few minutes that were actually just told to her.

I have worked with Alicia over the past couple of years giving her practice in recalling things to help her be better at using her short-term memory. Here is a typical example. I would say, "We need to go to the bank to make a deposit and then go to the grocery store." We would get in the car, and then a few minutes later, she would ask me, "So, where are we going?" When that happens, my first instinct was to feel like she was just kidding. When I realized that she did not remember, I would just wait until we got to the bank, and she would almost always then remember once she saw the bank. She'd say, "Oh, we're going to the bank to make a deposit and then to the grocery store."

I believe that she knew somewhere in her brain that we were going to the bank and the grocery store. The memory was there. However, the connection to the memory was interrupted. Once she had a familiar reference, in this case the sign in front of the bank, the connection to the memory was reestablished and the memory easily recalled.

Just as the result with the physical therapy, the speech therapist told Alicia that she did not need to come back any longer after four of five sessions. She told Alicia, "There isn't much more I can do for you. You need to go home and let us deal with patients with more serious conditions."

What I think anyone dealing with a family member recovering from a stroke needs to remember is that progress is made in baby steps, not in gigantic improvements all at once. In some areas, you will see rapid improvement. However, in other areas you might not see any improvement for a number of weeks or months. The changes are subtle or unnoticeable from one day to the next. You will see some improvement in one area. Then, there does not appear to be any more progress in that area for a while. And, then, later you will notice improvement again, often when you least expect it.

It is a challenge to know whether any further improvement is possible in the area which has plateaued. In our case, I would give Alicia around three months of a plateau in any one area before I would begin to think that the plateau is the final result. I experienced a number of areas that would plateau for weeks only to improve again. I go into more detail about this in Chapter 12.

I think it is important to remember that improvements are made in all areas, not just mentally. Alicia was able to benefit from taking Pilates lessons that helped her improve her core muscle strength. I would recommend to anyone who is dealing with a family member of loved one who is recovering from a stroke that they deal with the recovery of the whole person – physically, mentally and spiritually. Improvement in one area affects the state of the others. You will see evidence of that in the remaining chapters.

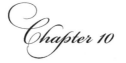

Chapter 10

BACK IN THE SADDLE AGAIN

"Whoopi-ty-aye-oh
Rockin' to and fro
Back in the saddle again
Whoopi-ty-aye-yay
I go my way
Back in the saddle again"

Gene Autry & Ray Whitley, *Back in the Saddle Again*
Reprinted by permission.

Background

One of the things Alicia has enjoyed doing most of her life is riding horses. She began by riding a neighbor's horse when she was eight years old. She got serious in high school. Her interest quickly focused on Hunter Jumper where the horse and rider go over a series of 2 ½ to 3 ½ foot jumps and are rated by a judge on how well they perform (against the perfect rider/horse).

Anyone who thinks this is easy to do should try it. It is very difficult to train the horse to follow the commands of the rider so that they can both approach the fence and jump it together such that the rider does not fall off or the horse does not hit the fence. After all, the horse cannot see the rider. They can only hear and sense commands from pressure of the rider's legs against the side of the horse.

Alicia progressed in her riding and when she was twelve years old, she begged her family to buy her a horse. Alicia's parents finally relented and bought Alicia her first horse named Sky Parade. It was purchased from Leak Kennedy in Atlanta where Alicia lived for $1,000 for her thirteenth birthday in September 1956. See Figure 10-1.

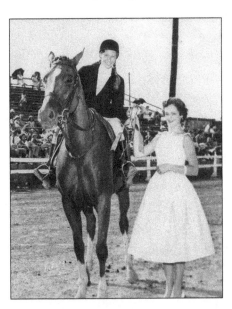

Figure 10-1. Alicia Grant riding Sky Parade (barn name 'The Mare') winning first place in the Henderson, NC horse show, Equitation Class, 13 and Under (September 1956).

In riding, an owners typically give his or her horse two names: a barn name for what the owner calls the horse around the barn during practice and a show name that is used only in the ring during competition. These names are typically one to three words. One of my favorites is "Daddy's Last Dollar." Alicia referred to her horse as "The

Mare" around the barn. When introduced at horse shows, the horse was referred to by her show name, e.g. "Next in the ring is Sky Parade owned and ridden by Alicia Grant."

Alicia began riding almost every day at Fritz Orr, a riding stable on Nancy Creek Road near her house on Ridgewood Road. Fritz Orr's property is now part of The Westminster Schools and has become the practice field for the football team.

Leak gave Alicia riding lessons and helped her qualify to compete in Hunter show classes in local horse shows. Alicia rode locally in Atlanta and participated in some fox hunting events as well. Alicia started to compete in horse shows first at Chastain Park in Atlanta but soon began traveling to other horse shows around the Southeast. She won her first Equitation Hunter class in Hendersonville, NC on Sky Parade in 1956 (see Figure 10-1).

After a few years, Sky Parade developed some problems and began to refuse jumps. Consequently, Alicia had to give her away.

In 1960 when Alicia was 17, the family leased Dig's Frills from Mickey Baker. He had two horses for sale: Dig's Frills and Lady Luck. Alicia tried both of them, and Alicia really loved Dig's Frills, but her parents did not buy either one of them. Her dad sent Dig's Frills back to Mickey Baker because the horse had a club foot even though he jumped well. Alicia wanted Dig's but her dad did not want to take the risk.

Alicia talked with Mickey, and he agreed to lend her their second horse, Lady Luck, but she was not a competitive horse. Finally, after spending time on Lady Luck, Alicia told Mickey she really wanted to ride Dig's Frills. Mickey agreed to swap Lady Luck for Digs, but he would not let Alicia's family buy her. She enjoyed riding Digs and won a number of major classes including a popular show in Blowing Rock, NC (see Figure 10-2). She continued riding at the University of Georgia in the early 1960s but eventually gave it up when she started to work and have children.

Alicia started riding again in 1988 as her children got older. In more recent years, Alicia got back to serious riding in the hunter classes.

Cathy Whiteside became her trainer in Atlanta and Sandy Ferrell her trainer during the winter season in the Winter Equestrian Festival in Wellington, Florida which is the equestrian capital of the world from January through the end of March. Riders come from all over the world to enjoy the mild weather and compete in Dressage (rated but no jumping), Hunter (jumping and rated) and Jumper (jumping and timed but not rated). The Hunter category is intended to encourage riders to learn how to jump over fences with the right form rather than going as fast as they can.

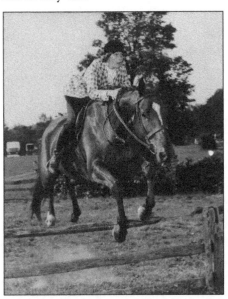

Figure 10-2. Alicia Grant riding Digs Frills (barn Name "Digs") at the Blowing Rock, NC horse show in 1960 at age 17. Note there are no "break-away" fences – scary!

Alicia owned a very athletic horse named Niles (show name "Champagne Country"). She was able to ride in the top amateur class called Amateur Owner over 3' 6" fences (see Figure 10-3). Unfortunately, in 2009, Niles threw Alicia off a number of times clearly indicating to

Alicia that he did not want to be in the ring jumping any longer. This change was right after horse had a serious infection called Lymphangitis that required extensive treatments. We think that the infection caused a permanent change in the horse's ability to jump. Alicia decided to donate Niles in March 2010 to Morrisville College, New York which has an extensive equestrian program.

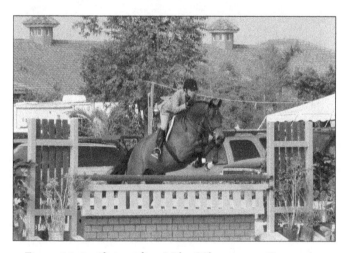

Figure 10-3. Alicia riding Niles (Champagne Country) in the Littlewood Horse Show, January 2007 – Amateur Owner Division at 3' 6" over fences.

Alicia was at a bit of a crossroad in riding. She did not have a horse and was not sure where to ride. She tried a few horses in Wellington before we returned to the Atlanta area in April 2010. She was not able to find another horse that she liked.

After returning to Atlanta in the spring of 2010, Cathy Whiteside mentioned that one of her clients, and, as it turns out, a long-time friend Barbara Goldsmith had a horse named Greta that might be available. Barbara was recovering from a heart procedure and offered to let Alicia ride her horse Greta (show name "Riesling"). As a consequence, Alicia rode at the Goldsmith's during the summer and fall of 2010. See Figure 10-4.

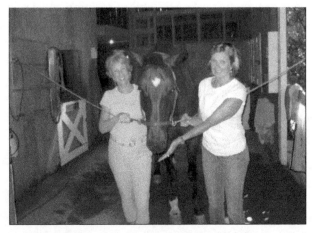

Figure 10-4. Alicia with her trainer Cathy Whiteside with Greta at Barbara Goldsmith's barn in Atlanta (August 2010). Cathy helped Alicia get back in the saddle on September 12, 2011.

Because Barbara had to have a second heart procedure, she offered to let Alicia take Greta for the 2011 winter season in Wellington. Alicia met with John Roper and Kelly Mullin who were training other riders (Wendy Gifford, Amy Smith, Joni Werthan and Julie Bush) at Canterbury Farm in Grand Prix Village in Wellington, Florida. John agreed to become her primary trainer and Kelly would do warm-ups and supplemental training when John was out of town judging other horse shows.

Fortunately, Barbara regained her health in 2011 so Greta was returned to the Goldsmith stables in March, but Barbara allowed Alicia to ride Greta a couple of times a week and take an occasional lesson from Cathy Whiteside. Alicia felt this was an interim situation that would allow her to find another horse to own or lease on a longer term basis.

Then, bam, Alicia had the stroke on August 23 and the future of her riding was put completely up in the air.

After her stoke in August 2011, Alicia shared that she was not sure whether she could ever ride again. Her left side was still a bit compromised, and she had to work on re-learning fine motor skills. But, she loved riding so much that she wanted to get back into riding as soon as possible. Because she made such a rapid recovery from physical therapy in the month following the stroke, Alicia called Cathy and asked her if she could help her get back into the saddle. Cathy agreed. On September 12, 2011, Alicia met Cathy at the Goldsmith's barn to assess the situation and see if Alicia might be able to ride again.

That first day was a bit stressful for Cathy and Alicia because neither one knew how it would go. While Alicia knew how to ride from fifty plus years of development of her riding skills (complying with Malcom Gladwell's 10,000 hours of practice to succeed at an activity in life in his famous book, Outliers), neither one of them knew how much her riding ability was compromised due to the stroke.

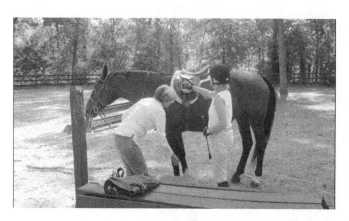

Figure 10-5. September 12, 2011 – Alicia about to get up on Greta at the Goldsmith's riding ring in Atlanta. This is her first time on a horse since her stroke. Would she stay up or fall off?

We all discussed the situation and realized that even if some of her skills were impaired, there was a very good chance that she could get back to riding successfully again by simply retraining her brain to control Alicia's movements to give proper signals to the horse. In other words, her brain had stored the knowledge and experience on how to ride, but she might need to train pathways to her muscles to tell them exactly what to do. See Figure 10-5.

I remember standing in the ring with Cathy, Alicia and Greta holding the reins while Cathy helped Alicia up the short step stool used by riders to get on a horse. We did not know if Alicia would jump up into the saddle like she did before or fall off the other side, or whether she would be able to jump up and sit in the saddle.

Cathy said, "OK, let's just get up and sit in the saddle at first to make sure you're comfortable doing that." With a "1-2-3," up Alicia went putting her right leg over the horse and sat in the saddle just like she always did. That worked out just fine. I'll never forget the big smile

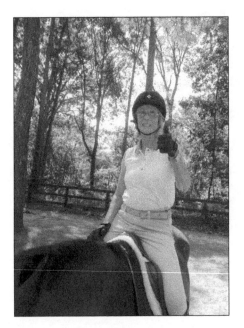

Figure 10-6. Alicia gives a thumbs up while riding Greta at Barbara Goldsmith's barn September 12, 2011. She was not at full strength but her history of riding horses helped her to get back to riding and enjoying life again.

Alicia had on her face as she was "back in the saddle again" for the first time since her stroke. I had a swelling in my throat over it because it meant that she could ride again – doing something she has enjoyed doing for most of her life. There was a rather big sigh of relief by all.

Cathy gave her the reins and suggested she just walk around the ring a few times to get used to basic walking movement. You would think that Alicia was a little girl riding for the first time. I mean, she was doing something that she knew how to do in her sleep, but it seemed amazing to see her doing it again. Alicia and Cathy were not sure what was going to happen, so both of them were pleased that it looked just like always. I was very proud of her.

Next, Cathy asked Alicia to get Alicia to go to the next level and give commands to Greta to trot. This is a bit more complex, especially for Alicia because she had to move up and down in the saddle in a rhythmic movement called "posting" while the horse is moving. Alicia had a bit of a problem getting Greta to move from the walk into a trot owing to her lack of strength in her legs, partly due to the stroke but also partly from not riding much for a few months prior to her stroke. See Figure 10-6.

I could see Alicia pressing her stirrups against Greta's side but the signal Greta was feeling clearly was not like it was before the stroke. Cathy told Alicia, "Squeeze harder!" and, sure enough, Greta began to trot, and Alicia proceeded to post by rising up and down in the saddle. It was a little slow and Greta would return to a walk after a few seconds.

Alicia tried trotting with posting three or four times, and slowly I could see Alicia retraining the commands through her left leg. It became most noticeable was when Alicia was going counter-clockwise in the ring. When going counter-clockwise, Alicia had to press more with her left leg to keep the horse going right instead of left. Think about it: if you were the horse and could not see the rider, you would need to be told which way to go.

If someone pushed you on your left side, you would move to the right to get away from the pushing. This is the same process a rider uses to tell the horse which direction to go. Most of the control commands from the rider to the horse are through squeezing the legs and tapping or kicking with the rider's heals with a little fine adjustment from the tightness or direction of the reins.

Overall, Alicia's session on Greta overseen by Cathy Whiteside was considered a success. She was not yet able to get the horse to go faster (canter), but Alicia was confident that with some more experience riding, she would be able to control her horse as she did in the past.

As Barbara Goldsmith continued to recover from her heart condition, she naturally wanted to spend more time with her horse. Plus, Adrian Berry, daughter of Dr. Currell Berry, also had a horse at the Goldsmith's barn. She was now riding more seriously and was taking lessons from Cathy Whiteside at the Goldsmith's barn. As a result of this, Alicia realized that she was not going to be able to take Greta back to Florida for the next winter season as she had done from January to April 2011.

As a result, Alicia had two challenges. First, Alicia had to find a new horse, and she also had to find another place ride during the summer when we were back in Atlanta. While Wellington is a wonderful place to live, the equestrian community leaves by mid-April thus making it almost impossible to ride with professional trainers during the summer months. And, in addition to all that, all the major horse shows are outside of Florida. As the weather gets warmer, the horse shows move north.

Alicia's good friend Peggy Knight mentioned that she had a half lease of a horse named Abbey at New Vintage Farm (NVF) in Woodstock, GA (north of Atlanta and west of Alpharetta). NVF is owned by Julie Curtin whom Alicia knew casually from being around the horse show circuit for years.

Peggy asked Julie if Alicia could come out and visit NVF and do a test ride on Abbey with Julie giving supervision. Peggy told Julie that Alicia had had a stroke but was getting back into riding. Julie later shared that she thought, "Oh dear, I've got a stroke victim who wants to take riding lessons. I wonder if she can stay on the horse?"

Alicia and I went out to New Vintage Farm on December 17, 2011 to meet Julie and take a practice ride on Abbey. There were really a number of objectives for this meeting and riding session: 1) let Julie have an assessment of Alicia's post-stroke skill, 2) check out Abbey as a horse possibly to ride when we were in Atlanta, 3) evaluate New Vintage Farm as place in which to ride after the winter season in Wellington and 4) let Alicia continue to practice her equestrian skills. See Figure 10-7.

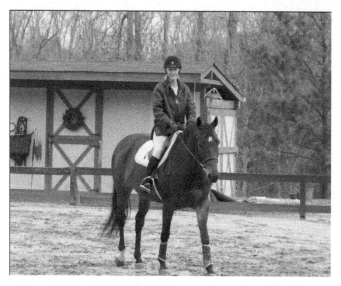

Figure 10-7. Alicia riding Abbey on December 24, 2011 at New Vintage Farm. Abbey is owned by Emily Kleinberg who was away at college. This was a temporary riding arrangement until Alicia returned to Wellington where her winter trainer, John Roper, told Alicia he would find her a new horse.

Alicia really enjoyed riding Abbey. She was very impressed with Julie's training skills and felt Julie would be great trainer during the summer months when we lived in Atlanta Alicia also liked New Vintage Farm and Julie Curtin (Figure 10-8).

There were around forty horses and stalls at New Vintage Farm which meant that there would likely always be other riders there when Alicia was riding. Also, Julie often took groups of riders to various horse shows in nearby locations like Conyers, Wills Park, Aiken, SC, Blowing Rock, NC, Fairburn and the Brownland Horse Show in Franklin, TN (near where Alicia's youngest daughter lives).

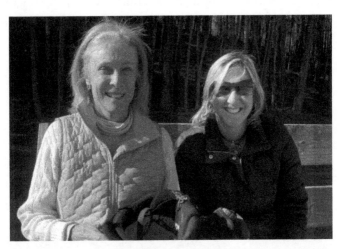

Figure 10-8. Alicia with her new trainer, Julie Curtin, of New Vintage Farm. Photo taken at New Vintage Farm on December 17, 2011 after Alicia had practiced riding Abbey.

Julie did a great job working with Alicia. As she said, "When Alicia took her first lesson with me, the main concern that popped into my mind was safety. Because I am a fellow rider, I know the overwhelming love and dedication that riding brings. These emotions can be overwhelming.

"My main goal for the first lesson was to provide a safe environment with a trusting mount that Alicia could feel comfortable with in hopes that some of the joy and familiarity of riding could return. Since Alicia had been riding for a major part of her life, I was hoping that her body would remember the familiar movements associated with taking the horse over a jump. Sure enough, with a trusty mount Alicia was able to jump again looking confident and in control."

Alicia loved being back in the saddle again. She felt that Julie was just the kind of trainer she needed to help her get over the anxiety of riding and jumping again. Just before we migrated to Wellington for the winter season, Alicia asked Julie if she would be willing to be her trainer after the Winter Equestrian Festival was over in April. Julie told Alicia that she would be delighted to have her at NVF. [Note: the barn at New Vintage Farm burned to the ground on Thanksgiving morning November 26, 2014. Julie installed a circus tent while the barn was rebuilt and reopened in the spring of 2016.]

While Alicia felt that Julie and NVF were great, her temporary riding companion Abbey was not a horse in which she could ride at the competition level required in Wellington, which involved riding against the best riders in the country during the winter season.

Alicia called her winter trainer John Roper who lives in Franklin, Tennessee and asked him if he thought he could find a good, safe horse but one that would enable Alicia to be competitive in the Winter Equestrian Festival.

When we relocated to Wellington after Christmas, Alicia was in touch with John frequently. In the first week of January 2012, John told Alicia that he had found a good prospective horse called Polina that was owned by Carlie Newwonder and was stalled with Alan Korotkin and Susan Tuccinardi at Castlewood Farm in Wellington. Polina was a bit older (18) but had won many classes. In other words, she had good blood lines and had a good track record competing in Hunter classes. She was also solid and safe.

John Roper, Alicia and I went over to Castlewood Farm (Figure 10-9) to take a look at Polina. John and Alicia took the prospective horse, Polina, out to their ring. Alicia got up with John watching over her. After she went around the ring a couple of times, John asked her what he thought, and Alicia blurted out, "John, I love this horse. She is just perfect. I can tell. I want to ride this horse!"

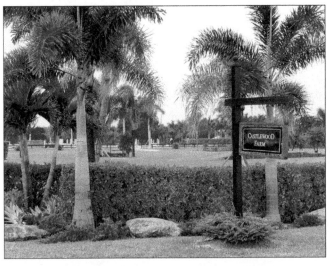

Figure 10-9. Castlewood Farm in Wellington, Florida, where John Roper found Polina in January 2012 for Alicia to ride (and where Alicia would later ride Ella).

John then arranged to have Polina sent over by trailer from Castlewood Farms to Canterbury Farm since it was a couple of miles away. See a photo of Canterbury Farm Figure 10-10.

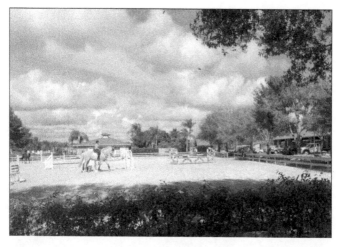

Figure 10-10. Beautiful Canterbury Farm practice ring in Grand Prix Village, Wellington, Florida where Alicia rode each day before competing in the Winter Equestrian Festival.

John had input from Julie Curtin that Alicia was making progress in her post-stroke recovery, but that her strength was still not back to normal, particularly on her left side. Going around the ring counter-clockwise was more difficult for Alicia since it required her to provide constant pressure with her left, more compromised leg. See Figure 10-11 with John, Alicia and her new horse, Polina.

Alicia also had some difficulty giving Polina a strong enough command to go quickly from a walk directly to a canter. The canter is a controlled, three-beat gait that is like a gallop only a bit slower and more controlled. Alicia could easily get Polina to trot but going from walk to cantor was more challenging. John had to spend some time working with Alicia on strengthening her left leg and practicing going from the walk to a canter many times. John got a bit frustrated. One time, he reached down, picked up some sand in the ring and threw it at Polina's rear end to help get her to canter. We have since laughed about that event at many group dinners.

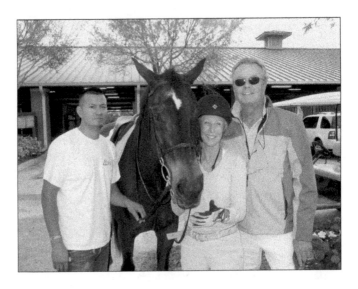

Figure 10-11. Alicia with her trainer, John Roper, and her groom (Chris) as well as with her new horse Polina (January 29, 2012) at Canterbury Farm in Grand Prix Village.

Kelly Mullen sometimes rode Polina to give her full commands, to get her ready to jump over fences and to train her when Alicia and I were out of town. Kelly has become a good friend along with John. They operate separate businesses regarding clients. In Alicia's case, Alicia needed to have Polina get some supplemental riding from a professional trainer. Since John does not any longer ride, Kelly rode Polina both to warm her up and to give Polina a reference on what Kelly wanted the horse to do going over the various jumps.

Sometimes when the riding lessons began, Alicia would have a difficult time with a particular movement, e.g. doing figure eight's or timing the jumps correctly. Consequently, Kelly would ride Polina for five minutes going around commanding her more intensely than Alicia was able to do to remind Polina what she is supposed to do. Then, Alicia would get back on Polina. The horse would be tuned and able to accept Alicia's similar but less intense commands to do the same thing. At other times, Kelly would come out early and warm up Polina, particularly on the morning of a day in which Alicia would be riding in the horse show. Kelly would get Polina warmed up and ready to go in the ring. See Alicia riding Polina during a training session at Canterbury Farms (Figure 10-12).

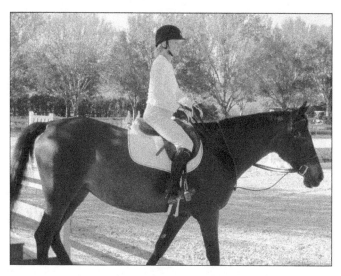

Figure 10-12. Alicia riding Polina in the practice ring in Canterbury Farm in Grand Prix Village in early 2012 after just getting Polina.

Alicia made very good progress starting in January 2012. She improved each week until the end of February when John felt Alicia had regained enough strength and head relearned how to control the horse in a horse show where she would have to jump a series of seven or eight jumps in the right sequence.

Alicia's first time back in the ring was February 23, 2012 (Figure 10-13). One of the things that is most difficult to regain following a stroke is multi-tasking or, in Alicia's case, the ability to control the horse

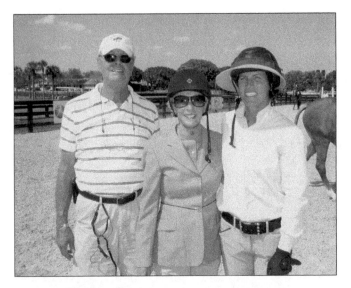

Figure 10-13. John Roper, Alicia Purdy and Kelly Mullen on February 23, 2012. This was the first time Alicia competed in a horse show following the stroke in August 2011.

to do the jumps in the right sequence with just the right timing and to remember the order of the jumps. Remembering the order of the jumps is one thing that has continued to be difficult for Alicia. .

One time in March 2012 Alicia and John went over the jump sequence for the class in which she was showing. He had her repeat the sequence aloud to him at least two times. Alicia would say something like this, "OK, I go in and do a left lead (where the horse leads its stride with the left leg versus the right leg). Then I jump the single oxer (two poles side by side that makes the jump a bit longer than a single pole) and then do the inside six (meaning that that the horse is to take exactly six strides from the first jump to the second jump). Then, I do the outside five (five strides between two jumps set up along the outside of the ring). Then, I come back the other diagonal in seven and end up over the single jump toward the entry gate."

I am sure most anyone reading this will think that it is very difficult to remember to do Hunter classes. You are right. It takes years of riding to get the feel for the horse so that you know how to lead the horse into the jump in a way that the horse will not take off too far away (called "unseating the rider" or "being left") or too close to the jump which often causes the horse to take an extra stride (called a "chip"). Each rider is being judged as to how well she is able to command the horse during the series of jumps as it takes a lot of skill to command the horse to do the jumps correctly.

A rider in the Hunter class is in the ring for typically about two minutes, but during that short time, the rider and the horse are going about fifteen miles an hour while timing the approach correctly so that the horse goes over each jump at the right time forming a nice well balanced arc on both sides jump and keeping the horse in the middle of the jump. Doing a complete round in the ring is, therefore, very challenging and requires great multi-tasking skills. I have to admit that I am extremely proud of Alicia's being able to practice an hour every day, to have the strength to do this and to get back the skills she developed over the past fifty plus years in order to ride her horse in a competitive horse show.

In a typical show, Alicia would do a warm-up rounds on Thursday. Some of these rounds are what's called a "ticketed warm-up" where the rider is doing the jumps in the same sequence as in the real judged class but no judge is there. Then, she will ride in official classes against thirty to fifty other riders on Friday, Saturday and Sunday with an extra "Under Saddle" class thrown in for good measure. In the Under Saddle class (also called the "hack" class), the horse and rider walk, trot and canter in front of the judge to see which horse has the best gait. It takes a lot of experience as a judge to sort through the different horses since they are all doing the same thing.

Alicia's hard work paid off handsomely for her. On March 2, 2012. She competed in the Low Adult Hunter class and won first place. See Figure 10-14. This event was a major moment in her recovery from her stroke six months prior. We honestly did not know if Alicia could return to her previous skill level which had enabled her to successfully compete against thirty plus other riders in the thirty-five and older Adult Hunter division.

Alicia was able to do all of the jumps in the sequence correctly without a mistake, and because it was the Winter Equestrian Festival, she had to do those jumps better than fifty plus other riders representing the best in the United States. Riding is a sport where you can compete until well into your seventies if you are able to stay healthy, workout regularly, have a good horse and, of course, have a good trainer. It all came together for Alicia that day. There are so many variables in

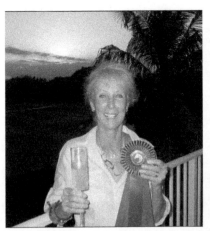 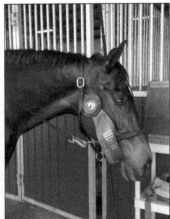

Figure 10-14. Alicia winning first place in the Low Amateur Adult hunter on March 2, 2012. Photo taken on our balcony overlooking the golf course at sunset. Second photo shows Alicia's horse Polina with the blue ribbon.

competitive riding that makes it difficult for anyone, even those who spend hundreds of thousands of dollars on a world-class horse, to compete and win regularly.

On the other hand, things can easily come unraveled when in the show ring. One day in March 2012, Alicia competed in the 2' 6" Adult Low Adult Hunter class. It was raining, but the temperature was quite warm in the high 70s. She did the round perfectly. We were all excited that she was going to get a good, high ribbon.

Then, instead of doing a slow circle to cool down and exit the ring, she kept going. At first, I thought she was just making a bigger circle to cool off, but I could quickly tell she was starting to do the course a second time without stopping! I said, "Alicia, I don't think you're supposed to be doing that." Then, I said, "Stop! You're finished! Alicia! Stop! Alicia, don't do those jumps again!"

Her trainer John Roper said something like, "What in the world is Alicia doing?" Finally, the announcer came over the PA with "Polina is off course – you're excused – thank you". That is a very nice way of saying you messed up big time and that you were eliminated from the class.

Alicia later said, "Well, I wasn't sure if I had done all the jumps, so I thought I'd keep going until something inside told me it was over." This is both terribly funny (we all laughed when we got together about her doing the course a second time), but it also points out the challenge of totally recovering from a stroke. Multi-tasking requires the brain to do many things correctly all at the same time. The demands are great. When there's a permanent impairment such as Alicia had from the stroke where millions of neurons and axons in her brain died during the gap between finding the clot and removing it, a lot of time and numerous repetitive exercises are required to relearn multi-tasking in order to prevent any mistakes in the ring.

It seems at times that this particularly high demand on Alicia's brain might not totally return. All riders forget their course at one time or another. It happens to everyone. It appears at this point two years after her stroke that memorizing the course in the show ring is still challenging because of the demands on her short-term memory and multi-tasking.

Alicia gets the course right almost all the time now, but it takes some effort. She verbalizes the course to her trainer, looks at the course from different perspectives and imagines going over the jumps. In a typical class, the sequence is to do a line to the outside of the ring followed by a diagonal line on the inside and returning to the outside. Knowing that the lines alternate is helpful because if the rider has just done an inside diagonal, they that rider knows that the next line will be on the outside of the ring.

Trainers typically refer to the lines by the number of strides that are required to be performed. Most of the time, the distance between the jumps in a hunter class results in either four, five, six or sometimes seven strides. The trainer will say something like, "OK you go do the outside five, followed by the inside seven and return to an outside single and then finish coming back with an inside six."

Once Alicia feels comfortable with the jump sequence, she is just like her old self when she gets in the ring. Then, it is a matter of execution: – getting the horse in the right position for each jump, coming off the jumps and moving forward quickly to make the second jump in the correct number of strides. When she executes well, she almost always gets a ribbon (one of the top eight horses in a class) and occasionally wins the class.

I suspect that the some of the other riders in a class know that Alicia had a stroke. They also know that she is one of the best amateur riders over fifty years old. When she executes her course in the right sequence, she is often going to be "the ribbons." She can be a bit intimidating to other riders as in, "How in hell does she do that? She's had a stroke for Pete's sake."

But, the opposite can occur as well. Even if Alicia completes the course without making any major mistake, it is possible that she still will not win. The competition at the Winter Equestrian Festival is the best to be found in one place in the entire country. Sometimes, you need to have perfect form over every single jump, not just to complete the course without making any mistakes, in order to be judged good enough to earn one of the ribbons.

There is one other award that riders in hunter classes can win: the Championship for their division. This is determined by points earned in the respective classes. One weekend day may have three classes (two hunter and one hack) while another day may just be two hunter classes.

The judge keeps a numerical score for each horse's performance based on how well the rider commanded the horse. Scores range from the low forties (when horse knocks down a rail or refuses a jump) up to the seventies for a good round, eighties for a great round and, rarely, in the low nineties for a near perfect round. If a rider places well in the day's competition, that rider may have a shot at the two awards given out for the overall best performances: Championship (highest total score) and Reserve (second highest score).

Alicia competed in a few shows during 2012 after leaving Wellington in April. One of her favorite horse show is the Brownland Horse Show in Franklin, TN. On Sunday, October 26, 2012, Alicia was having a good day guided by her trainer Julie Curtin. She won first place in one hunter class and second in the other class. We waited around to see if she might be in the running for Championship or Reserve, and sure enough, Alicia's total score was the highest so she won the Championship ribbon! That is a real honor since it is difficult to get either two wins out of three or to win everything against good competition.

The following photo (Figure 10-15) was taken as we were getting ready to leave the Brownland Horse Show and head back to our Atlanta area home. Julie came by to congratulate Alicia on her fine performance. I quickly took a very spur of the moment photo. You can feel how excited both of them were over this special win. This represented another testament that Alicia was able to make a full recovery from her stroke.

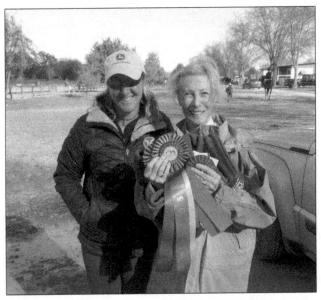

Figure 10-15. Alicia's trainer, Julie Curtin, with Alicia on Sunday, October 10, 2012 after Alicia has just won the Championship ribbon by winning a first and second place in the Low Adult Hunter division. This was her first Championship win since her stroke.

Now, take a look at the Figure 10-16. It was taken in Rost Arena at the Winter Equestrian Festival (WEF) on March 16, 2012. Alicia had a good round without making any mistakes. But, she did not win the class. She was very happy with this round even if she did not win. Another rider and horse simply did a little bit better. Try to imagine yourself in this photo and all the years of riding it took to develop the skill to jump as beautifully as Alicia did. But, Alicia always says, "When you have a great day riding, you're happy whether or not you win the first place blue ribbon."

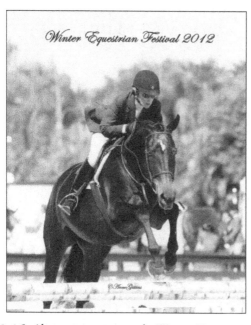

Figure 10-16. Alicia competing in the Winter Equestrian Festival, March 16, 2012 riding in the Rost arena (courtesy Anne Gittings).

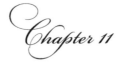

Chapter 11

TRYING TO FIGURE OUT
WHAT HAPPENED

"I wanna thank you very much
Thank for lending me love
Now I'm levitating
Cos I feel like I've been waiting
For a lifetime
For your love"

Westlife, *Thank You*
Reprinted by permission.

After having a stroke and then recovering from it, you wonder, "What in the world caused the stroke to happen?" Answering the first question then begs to ask a second question, "What can be done to prevent it from happening again?"

A lot of personal and medical systems efforts have gone in to answering these questions about Alicia's stroke. Clearly, *something* caused the clot to form and end up in the base of Alicia's brain. It certainly did not happen locally: no clot formed in Alicia's brain. Clots can form in the brain if there is previously some hemorrhaging from a rupture in the brain's arteries that leads to bleeding. In Alicia's case, she did not have any ruptured blood vessels.

A stroke caused by hemorrhaging in the brain is treated differently from the more frequent stroke that results from a clot formed elsewhere in the body which then travels to the brain down smaller and smaller arteries until it becomes lodged in a small crevice where it cannot go any further. The first thing to determine is the place of origin of the clot. Most of the time, perhaps as much as ninety percent of the time, clots are formed in the heart usually resulting from a heart arrhythmia, an abnormal heart beating sequence. This becomes the "smoking gun" for the cause of the stroke.

A common heart arrhythmia is atrial fibrillation that occurs in one of the two atria that feed blood into the two main pumping ventricles. The right ventricle pumps blood to the lungs to obtain oxygen and the left ventricle pumps blood to the rest of the body to service demands. Often, one of the atria can generate extra beats called a premature atrial contraction (PAC), but if those continue in rapid sequence, it can cause the atria to flutter and, as a result, the blood in the atrium doesn't move and begins to clot. A clot formed this way can subsequently travel from the atrium to the lung to form an embolism or to the brain to cause a stroke.

Even though the TEE procedure described in Chapter 5 did not isolate an existing clot in Alicia's heart, it was still most likely that the stroke-causing clot came from the heart. Therefore, once Alicia was discharged from the hospital, work began to focus on the heart as the most likely source of the clot. Our long-time family friend, Dr. Randy Martin, cardiologist at Piedmont Heart Institute in Atlanta and prior Assoc. Dean of Emory Medical School took over the investigation process. See Figure 11-1.

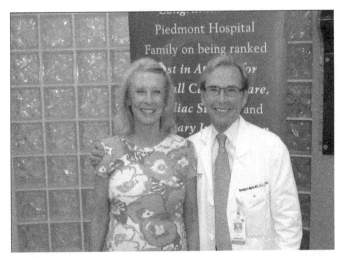

Piedmont Hospital
Family on being ranked
st in At   or
ll C   are,
liac S   and
ary

Figure 11-1. Alicia with Randy Martin, MD, FACC of the
Piedmont Heart Institute, Atlanta. Photo taken in the fall of
2011 while trying to determine what caused Alicia's stroke.

The first thing he did was to order a large battery of blood tests to
see if anything could be detected that might have caused the clot to form
that caused Alicia's stroke. Alicia went to the blood lab where they took
enough blood to fill approximately thirteen vials. Alicia asked the nurse
if they had left any blood for her.

The results of the blood tests were all negative: there were no
signatures of blood chemistry that provided the evidence to indicate
what had caused the clot to form. Thus, it appeared unlikely that
Alicia's blood chemistry itself had caused the clot that resulted in
the stroke.

The next avenue to pursue was whether she had any heart
arrhythmia that might have caused the clot. If Alicia had some
unknown occasional heart arrhythmia, this could be the cause of the
clot that triggered the stroke.

The process to determine if she had an occasional arrhythmia like atrial fibrillation was to wear a Holter Heart monitor for an extended time. Since it might be occurring only occasionally, Dr. Martin decided that Alicia should wear the monitor for a full month, both day and night. The only time it was taken off was when she took a shower. Here's a photo of a typical Holter monitor (Figure 11-2).

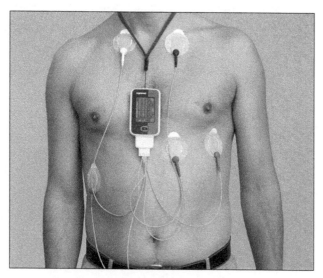

Figure 11-2. Typical Holter monitor setup with leads and radio transmitter.

Alicia and I worked together to get through this monitoring process. It was a bit uncomfortable having ECG leads stuck to Alicia's body all day and all night while she was trying to go about doing usual things. Because the leads were attached with an adhesive, we had to move them around slightly as they were changed each day to prevent irritation of the skin.

The Holter Monitor system has two main parts: 1) the leads and the Bluetooth transmitter and 2) the wide area wireless transmitter that is basically a custom-made, dedicated cell phone. The Bluetooth transmitter is a "'record and forward" device is powered by two AA batteries which had to be changed for new ones every couple of days. The wide area wireless transmitter is recharged overnight in a charging station that sits on the night stand.

Our routine was to change the ECG leads daily, charge the wide area wireless transmitter nightly and change the Bluetooth store and forward device every few days. In addition, we had to arrange the monitor using a belt clip so that Alicia could wear the entire system while she was riding her horse. Take a look at the next photo (Figure 11-3) where you can see the wide area wireless transmitter in the belt clip as it was attached to the rear of her riding outfit.

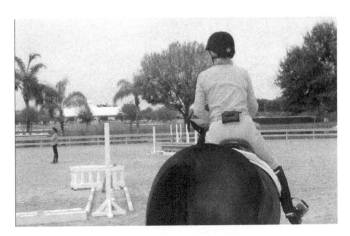

Figure 11-3. Alicia wearing the Holter monitor on January 29, 2012 while riding. Monitor was used for one month in an effort to determine what caused Alicia's stroke.

After wearing this for a month, the results were sent to Dr. Martin. He called to say that there were no arrhythmias detected the entire time Alicia wore the monitor. Therefore, Dr. Martin ruled out a *recurring* arrhythmia as the cause of the stroke.

Never the less, Dr. Martin felt that Alicia likely had a short bout of atrial fibrillation that caused the heart to briefly flutter. The arrhythmia allowed the blood to clot since it was not moving. The clot likely attached to the wall of the atrium and then dislodged on the evening of August 23, 2011 traveled up from the left ventricle through the right carotid artery and to the Medial Carotid Artery (MCA) where it came to rest in a very small artery that could not support the larger clot.

Now, this is where the story gets interesting (again) and likely brings to light what may have happened. It turns out that Alicia had two activities a few days before the onset of the stroke in which she was outdoors in high heat and humidity. She did not immediately recall that these two activities happened. Her recall came a number of months after the stroke.

Alicia and I believe one of these two outdoor activities put Alicia is a compromised position and gave new meaning to the words "heat stroke." Of course, just getting very hot from being outdoors does not typically cause a stroke. However, in Alicia's case, she certainly become over heated during both of these outdoor activities, and in at least one of them, she sensed that she experienced a "pounding heart" when she laid down to take a nap following both activities.

The first activity occurred on Thursday, August 18, 2011. Alicia enjoys playing tennis and wanted to have a tennis lesson. She went out to Bitsy Grant Tennis Center Thursday morning and had a tennis lesson. Because it was so hot in Atlanta ("Hotlanta"), the instructor did not have do a lot of running to hit the ball. However, even just standing in place for a thirty minute tennis lesson with the temperature in the mid-nineties can make any one over heated.

The second activity happened on Saturday, August 20, 2011, three days before Alicia suffered her stroke. She attended the Atlanta Summerfest horse show in Fairburn, Georgia just southwest of the Atlanta airport with her friend Peggy Knight. The temperature was well over ninety-five degrees that day, and Alicia was outside for more than six hours.

When she returned home after each of these outdoor activities in very hot weather, she was over-heated, dehydrated and exhausted so she took a nap. Alicia later remembered that during one of these naps, she woke up with her "heart pounding like mad." It subsided right after she woke up so she did not think anything of it. Alicia did not mention to me at the time that she had this pounding heart episode as she thought it was just from being overtired and over-heated. When she had the stroke, she temporarily lost the connection to that memory for a number of months.

One of the possible outcomes from doing the Holter monitor would be to find repeating atrial arrhythmias. If they were present, then Alicia would have to be put on a long-term blood thinner (like Warfarin/Coumadin, Xarelto or Eliquis) to reduce the likelihood of a clot forming from a future atrial arrhythmia event. However, since there were no recurring atrial (or other) arrhythmias present, it was decided that Alicia could just take an aspirin a day as well as maintain her post-stroke medication of Citalopram and Simvastatin that were prescribed when she left the hospital. This decision was particularly good news because it would have been difficult for Alicia to continue riding and face the risk of a problem occurring if she were to fall off the horse and suffer from uncontrolled bleeding.

Remember that a number of things improve after a stroke, and one of them is the memory around the time when the stroke occurred. A number of months later, Alicia suddenly recalled episode of having a pounding heart when she was napping following being outdoors and becoming over-heated. We discussed it with Dr. Martin. When Alicia laid down after those two outdoor activities and experienced a "pounding heart," she likely had a single bout of atrial fibrillation for a few minutes that caused a small clot to form in left side of her heart. It was attached to the wall of the left atrium or ventricle for three days until it dislodged around 6:30 pm on Tuesday, August 23, 2011 and, thus, caused the onset of the stroke.

Another possible aggravating factor may have been post-menopausal hormone replacement therapy (HRT). Alicia was taking HRT which can be a risk factor for strokes. Recall that Dr. Rivera and Dr. Frankel instructed Alicia to stop taking HRT as a result of her having a stroke since it could increase the likelihood of having another one. While there are no indicators that HRT caused the stroke, it might have contributed to the single bout of atrial fibrillation that occurred after one of the two outdoor activities a few days before Alicia suffered a stroke.

While we cannot prove with 100% certainty what caused Alicia's stroke, we believe it stemmed from her getting over-heated after one of these two outdoor activities.

That is the best guess at what we think happened. We may never know for sure but that seems to be the most plausible cause of Alicia's stroke.

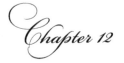

Chapter 12

A HEALTHY BUT SLIGHTLY DIFFERENT PERSON

"Days like these lead to...
Nights like this lead to
Love like ours.
You light the spark in my bonfire heart."

James Blunt, *Bonfire Heart*
Reprinted by permission.

Alicia has basically recovered to her full pre-stroke self with the primary exception of her intensity. I fortunately kept track of her progress as I noticed within the first month that her recovery was progressing at different rates for different attributes of her life. I kept track for over a year of the following traits she exhibited before the stroke:

1. Fine Motor Skills: doing things like putting in contact lenses, putting on a bracelet or watch or picking up small items. Alicia was completely normal regarding fine motor skills and, likely, a

bit better than most other people. She also had highly sensitive hearing. I often kidded her about being able to hear what the neighbors were talking about down the street.

2. Facial Control: control of the facial muscles especially when smiling. Alicia had normal facial muscle control before her stroke.

3. Equestrian: riding a horse and the degree of multi-tasking it requires. Alicia was an accomplished equestrian rider in the Hunter category for most of her life. Riding is something she did five or six days a week both for enjoyment, physical fitness and competition where she jumped her horse over fences 2' 6" or higher.

4. Spirituality: the sense of self as it relates to the universe and our creator, more than specifically affiliating with or going to a church. Alicia had always been one of the most spiritual persons I have ever known. She had tremendous "connections" and can sense things that many others cannot. She meditated daily and said her blessings and prayers.

5. Sexuality: the overall sexual response. Alicia was very typical before the stroke with a normal sexual response. We both enjoyed intimacy and loved each other every day, from kissing to hugging to holding each other while sleeping.

6. Multitasking: the ability to do multiple tasks at the same time. This is often the last area to return to normal after a stroke. Before her stroke, Alicia was a multitasking expert often doing lists of things or thinking of one thing while working on another. One of her favorite sayings was, "We've got to get organized." While all of us may have said that from time to time, Alicia would say it multiple times a day and then proceed to get whatever she was talking about organized and accomplished.

7. Painting: the ability to paint using watercolors or oils. Alicia was an accomplished artist using primarily oils. She painted an averaging around one painting every six months to a year.

8. Overall Intensity: how intense a person gets over various issues. Some people are very intense while others are more laid back. Before her stroke, Alicia was an intense person with strong views and feelings. She let you know where she stood and she could sometimes hold on to a feeling about something or someone for a very long time.

I put together a diagram that shows these eight aspects of Alicia's life. These are not golden nor would they be the same for another person, but they do represent Alicia well. In Figure 12-1 time is across the bottom from left to right representing the onset of the stroke to the end of 2012 or a total of around sixteen months. The percentage of full health is shown vertically on the left side from 0% (stroke level) to 100% of her pre-stroke level.

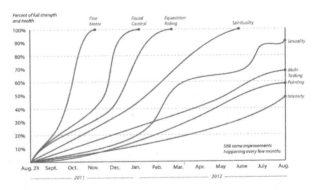

Figure 12-1. Diagram of Percentage back to full health vs. chronological time from onset of the stroke August 23, 2011 through 2012. Note that some of the traits recovered at different rates and took different recovery paths.

I have found most of these attributes have all returned to the pre-stroke 100% level with the exception of Alicia's intensity. I have described each of these traits in more detail below. In many cases, these attributes have been described earlier in other chapters. However, they are summarized here to help you visualize how these attributes changed over time.

Fine Motor Skills

One of the things that I noticed about Alicia's condition after she came home from the hospital was that a number of areas on her left side had been compromised in small ways. These were not the gross motor skills like moving an arm or leg, but, rather, a number of "fine motor skill" areas such as removing her contact lenses or picking up a spoon or knowing the feeling of where she put her left leg. I could see that these tasks could not be done exactly the same way they had been done before the stroke.

I mentioned earlier in detail how Alicia was having difficulty removing her contact lenses. When Alicia tried to take them out, she was having a very difficult time getting her fingers positioned correctly over the lens to pinch it and take it out. With my help, Alicia learned to reposition her fingers and retrain her brain so that subsequent efforts were successful.

Another example of the need to re-train an area controlled by fine motor skills was mentioned in detail in Chapter 9 – Rehabilitation. As I mentioned earlier, Alicia took a full three minutes more to do the task with her left hand than with her right. Over a period of a few weeks, Alicia was able to improve the time with her left hand to the point that there was little time difference between the time doing the task with her left and right hands.

It is truly amazing to watch the brain make adjustments and find new pathway to get something done. It is like witnessing the re-routing take place right in front of your eyes. Currently, Alicia does not have any compromised problems with fine motor skills. She still has a little bit of overall difference in the strength of her left side versus her right side, but her fine motor skills are back to normal.

Facial Control

The one thing that is noticeable right away in most anyone who has had a stroke is that facial expressions seem out of whack. Take a look at the following two photos: the one on the left is a photo of Alicia smiling before the stroke and the one on the right is a photo of her the day she came home from the hospital. The difference is striking, almost shocking.

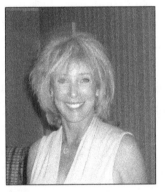 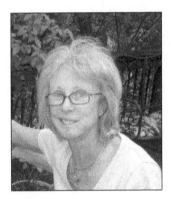

Figure 12-2. Alicia Purdy smiling before the stroke (left) and four days after the stroke (right). The uneven smile resulted from her being able to smile on her unaffected right side but unable to lift her facial muscles on her left side thus making the smile looks uneven.

The thing to note is that the stroke was on the right side of her brain, and, as a result, the lack of control was exhibited on the left side of her face. In many of Alicia's post stroke photos, however, it looks as if her right side is "off" when in fact her left side simply did not move to the extent that her right side moved. Hence, this made her smile look unbalanced.

It took Alicia about three months for her smile to return to normal. You can see in the photos from 2012 and in more recent ones that there is no longer any problem with Alicia's smile. A dramatic example is at the end of Chapter 13.

Equestrian/Riding

Alicia has ridden a horse since before she was ten years old so watching her riding skills progress was very interesting as they came back faster than I would have expected. We covered her equestrian development both before and after the stroke in Chapter 10 – Back in Saddle Again. What I want to point out here is her ability to ride came back quite quickly compared to a number of other attributes.

Alicia got back on a horse on Sept. 12, 2011 or just 20 days after the stroke. She did not ride again until December owing to a number of fall activities including a vacation trip to Hawaii in November and her needing to find a horse and a place in which to ride.

It was after we relocated to our home in Wellington right after Christmas that John Roper found the perfect horse for Alicia named Polina ("Polly" is her barn name). With significant training almost every day, Alicia was able to get back into show shape to compete in the Winter Equestrian Festival and win a number of top placing ribbons. I was extremely proud of her.

I also think that because Alicia had spent tens of thousands of hours riding, it was a core part of her being. She had developed many pathways in the brain to accomplish her riding. Although a few areas were compromised (predominantly on her left side), she had a number of ways to control the horse. Still, she had to work on building strength in her left leg. If Alicia took a break from riding for two to three weeks because of travel or other reasons, she had to take a couple of lessons to concentrate on using her left side muscles to give the correct signals to the horse.

Spirituality

Alicia has always been a spiritual person. She has a sense of things that are about to happen and she often can see things in others that most people ca not see. I remember before the stock market and real estate crash 2007, Alicia had a foreboding of black horses coming over a ridge. The stock market crashed right after that.

Both Alicia and I have read Power vs. Force by David Hawkins, MD. He has studied spirituality and human consciousness for many years. We were able to attend one of his day-long seminars in Sedona, Arizona before he passed away.

Alicia was able to achieve a high level of consciousness through her daily meditation. Although we do not go to church very often (mostly owing to the requirements of her equestrian program on Sunday mornings), we both discuss spirituality issues almost every day.

After Alicia had her stroke, she commented about having spiritual connections in her meditations and during her naps. I think her brain was in overdrive trying to make reconnections and at times reached a higher state of consciousness. Alicia never reported that she saw herself outside her body or approaching a tunnel with a bright light (as many report when they have had a near-death experience), but clearly there were a lot of connections going on both physically and spiritually.

It is interesting to note that during her recovery she felt spirits around her sometimes sitting on the bed or whirling around the room. Rather than ghosts, most of these spirits were energies with a warm, friendly and supportive vibe. I believe that people like Alicia have a brain that can capture interactions with spirits, like a fine tuned antenna. It is certain that highly spiritual people (Jesus, Mohammad, Dr. David Hawkins and many others) were able to meditate and sense things that exist in the universe that others cannot. Alicia has some of those qualities.

As a result, Alicia would report that she felt a presence. One evening about a month after the stroke as Alicia and I were getting ready to go to bed, she said she saw some spirits sitting on the end of the bed. They were not talking or trying to communicate but were simply there. She sensed a bit of discomfort from the spirts being there as if they were from beyond or the afterlife and that there was a reason for their presence. I felt them a couple of times myself at the same time she did and a couple of times in my downstairs office.

From what Alicia reported of her sense of their spirits, I think they were sent to visit and reassure her that she was not going to die, that she should know that God cared deeply about her and knew she was going to recover.

Also, about a year after Alicia suffered her stroke, she recalled that she did have a spiritual connection of some kind during her surgery to remove the blood clots in her brain. Again, the connection was not the "bright light" or "tunnel." Rather, it was more of a presence coming to her, not her going somewhere else. She felt the presence was there to reassure her that she would be OK.

Eben Alexander, MD in his popular 2012 book Proof of Heaven: A Neurosurgeon's Journey into the Afterlife, reported about his near death experience (NDE) while in a meningitis-induced coma in 2008. While Dr. Alexander's recollection included human figures, he also reported feeling spiritual presences, much like what Alicia recalled.

What seems clear is that Alicia's and Dr. Alexander's brains were put into very stressful, demanding situations. It seems that people may have an ability to interact with the universe in ways that are very special and unique when under extreme stress. Others who have trained their brains for many years can do similar things by their own command and control.

The message here to others is to be careful about how you react if someone close to you reports an unusual spiritual experience while recovering from a stroke. It is best to listen and let the stroke patient have multiple opportunities to discuss what happened. In Alicia's case, it seems to have been something that had more presence from the night of the stroke and then for about a year after. I believe she was able to report her experiences because of her meditating every day.

Sexuality

This is not going to be a <u>Fifty Shades of Gray</u> commentary, but sexuality is a part of all of our lives so it is important for everyone to know what to expect sexually after someone experiences a stroke. When Alicia came home from the hospital, she was clearly compromised and all energy was focused on taking care of her and helping her recover. Intimacy was experienced more in holding her at night and telling her how much I loved her.

I think the biggest thing to realize for any mate of a stroke victim is to understand that if their risk for a subsequent stroke is low, making love will not cause another stroke. Let me put this another way: strokes are not caused by a sexual experience. Rather, most are caused by atrial fibrillation that results in a clot being formed typically in the heart that subsequently travels to and gets lodged in the brain. If physical activity such as having sex is permitted following a stroke, that experience itself is not going to cause another stroke.

In spite of that, I personally felt very fearful that making love would cause another stroke. I think it is natural to feel that and, of course, some people could be in a "high risk" category for stroke reoccurrence, but in Alicia's case, this was a freak occurrence and the likelihood of reoccurrence was extremely low.

We waited until Alicia was feeling back to normal and then talked about it. I shared my fears and got encouragement from Alicia that she did not feel she would have another stroke. Thus, we entered the area of love making very slowly and very cautiously, taking it one step at a time. In retrospect, we were likely way too cautious, but we felt that going slow as the right choice.

As for Alicia, the primary thing I can report is that her recovery in sexuality was in phases or levels, not an all-at-once kind of response. So, anyone who has a loved one should realize that some of the pathways have to be relearned in the sexuality area just like relearning to take out your contact lenses.

The total recovery process was not smooth and linear like continually making one small improvement after another. Rather, it was one small improvement that lasted for weeks and then another improvement and then a few weeks later another improvement. The sexual recovery thus came in thresholds of recovery. But, with time, a full recovery in sexuality did come about, although it took over a year to achieve that.

We can say now that we are like honeymooners again. We do not even think about it as a recovery issue, but it did take a long time to reach that point. I hope that anyone reading this will better understand what to expect in this area. We had no previous knowledge in this area so we felt we were venturing into the unknown. The doctors did not discuss it, and we did not ask them about it. We did not find any references about post-stroke sexuality in books or online so we did not have any guidelines as a reference. But, we are happy that we took our time and that full recovery came about.

Multitasking

Clearly, multitasking was the most challenging area in which Alicia had to recover. It is hard to realize or understand what this means in practice. No one goes around every day thinking in terms of multitasking: you just do the things that you think are important. Before her stroke, Alicia was one of the best at planning, organizing and doing many things at the same time.

She had lists, and she kept a detailed calendar. She also had her friends with whom she talked all the time. It just felt natural. I admired her ability to be so organized. I am fairly organized myself, but it was a bit intimidating to have my wife more organized than I am. I had to keep up. "Gerry, did you get those three things done today?" Or, "I need to get organized to plan our trip to New York."

After the stroke, Alicia was the opposite of being organized. In fact, it was not until about six months later in the spring of 2012 that she said on her own, "We have to get organized" about something.

Now, that does not mean that Alicia was not able to get things done. She got a lot done. However, her immediate recovery was about going through rehabilitation at Northside Hospital and taking naps.

When we hired Genna Brown, the first thing we did was to use a large calendar to plan out short-term activities over the coming week or two. We helped Alicia plan, and we helped her get to an appointment or to a luncheon. However, she had lost a lot of her self-motivation to plan things herself. We talked about things that needed to get done. She understood them and could write them on the calendar, but it took many months for her to begin to plan things out for herself.

Realize that anyone recovering from a stroke will have a hard time with multitasking. They are most likely able to understand everything and agree that something is going to get done "next Friday" but it takes a while for them to say things like, "I think we need to plan out our schedule" or "I need to get these five things done today." You can tell someone recovering from a stroke something like, "Why don't you sit down and plan out what you want to get done today?" We did that often. In the beginning, Alicia would say things like "I don't know." It seemed like the little area of "planning self-motivation" had been zapped.

Slowly, however, Alicia began to plan things better. Improvement was in small increments but after about a year, she was able to function better in the planning area. She will sometimes need me to remind her of short-term activities. In fact, it seemed as if her long-term planning capability came back a lot faster than her short-term planning.

This is another important issue for someone recovering from a stroke: it takes years for some things like multi-tasking to make a full recovery. In fact, because improvements in multi-tasking take so long, it's easy to believe that the ability to multi-task just is not going to get any better. Even so, most people recovering from a stroke will improve over time. In some cases, it takes just months while in others it can take a year two. In Alicia's case, improvement in multi-tasking seemed to be like training for an athletic event: she had to train in order to be better at it, and if she stop training, she would fall back. But, she also had to train under direction so that the effort would enable repeating a task correctly. Training alone without proper instruction would be ineffective.

One must distinguish between short-term memory issues and multi-tasking. These two capabilities interact with each other, but they are different. Alicia might forget where we are going but once something is learned and put into longer term memory, then the recall is easier. Short-term memory can affect remembering the things that involve multi-tasking but by writing down the tasks, they become easier to remember later.

Remember that short-term memory lapses are lapses in the connection to the memory not necessarily the memory itself. This is very important. The brain stores the memory but sometimes loses the connection. Once the link is re-established, then the entire memory is recalled. In Alicia's case, she is able to remember things over the short–term (minutes) if she verbalizes the things she needs to remember. Verbalizing seems to work best for Alicia and reduces the loss of the link to the memory. Each time she has a short-term memory loss, I find it interesting that the entire memory comes back once she is reminded of the facts in the memory because the link gets reestablished and, thus, the details can be recalled.

Painting

Alicia is an accomplished artist. She has been drawing, doing watercolors and using oil paints to make some wonderful scenes (see www.aliciagpurdy.com). Before her stroke, Alicia averaged producing one serious oil painting a year plus a few other watercolor and sketches.

It was very interesting to watch Alicia get back into painting after her stroke. Her first attempt at doing a painting after the stroke was to do a fall tree that Alicia and I often see when walking around Chastain Park in North Atlanta. This tree becomes a very bright orange in late October. Alicia started by getting the overall shape correctly but it was missing a lot of detail. She would work on it from time to time and slowly, a great representation of the tree emerged from the canvas.

Take a look at the Figure 12-3. It shows a photo of the tree on the left and the painting of her representation of that tree on the right. In

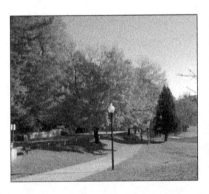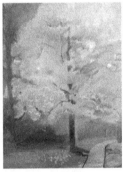

Figure 12-3. This is one of many beautiful fall trees in Chastain Park in North Atlanta. The tree turns very orange in the fall even though the top part is bare. Alicia's painting of this tree is shown on the right.

addition to referencing the photo, we also went out for walks where Alicia would look at the tree to get some ideas about how to represent it. She believes this is now about ninety percent done but plans to make a few more adjustments before she feels it is finished.

Here we are three years after her stroke, and she still does not spend the time painting the way she used to. She loves it when she does paint, but no longer paints most every day.

However, her long time and dear friend Jenny London has been responsible for helping Alicia get back into painting on a more regular basis. Alicia reached out to Jenny in the summer of 2013 as a way to find someone to share her painting experience. Jenny had recovered from breast cancer and was looking to paint more often also, as the two of them had done years ago. Alicia and Jenny now get together once every two to three weeks when we are in the Atlanta area. Here is a photo of the two of them painting at our house:

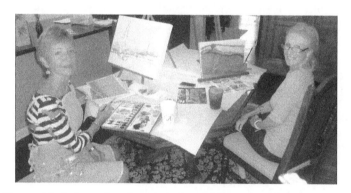

Figure 12-4. Jenny London and Alicia during one of their painting sessions at our home in the Atlanta area. They decided to both work on water colors in this session whereas they spend most of their sessions using oil paints. This process has been good for both of them – helping each of them recover from their prior affliction.

Overall Intensity

The final attribute that I tracked during the first year after Alicia's stroke was her intensity. This is a rather hard attribute to define but is one of those things that you know what it means without having a rigorous definition.

In this case, we're talking about the amount of energy spent on a given topic and the overall emotional attachment to it. Alicia has always been a focused person doing things in life with a vengeance. She does not just ride a horse. Rather, she rides her horse with the intent of winning every time she goes into the show ring. Alicia plans parties with the same intensity that are to die for: the food has to be great, the experience has to be wonderful for each guest, and she always wants to look fabulous.

Alicia is also very intense about finances. She was an auditor and credit manager at Bendix Corporation and knows how to budget and how to plan spending. When unexpected financial obligations come up that upset the budget, she got quite upset about it. Or, if we needed more money, she would say things like, "I need you to find another $3,000 this month to meet our obligations." She could be a tough task manager about financial things, but it is one of the reasons that she has managed her estate well. The values keep going up because she does not spend more than she makes.

Just about everyone who comes in contact with Alicia loves her dearly. She has a magnetic attraction in which she makes other people feel comfortable and good. There are more people who communicate with Alicia than any other person I know. I used to say that Alicia is the only person I know who exceeded the unlimited voice calling plan on her cell phone when mobile plans were based on talk time.

After the stroke, Alicia became much less intense. She would spend afternoons taking a nap or just lounging around. At first, this was very necessary to help her brain in recovering and working out alternate pathways around the damaged area. But after a year, I could see that she was not ever going to be as intense as before. I have kidded her that it is easier for me to live with her after the stroke as she does not get after me to do things like she did before the stroke.

Alicia has slowly regained her ability to oversee finances and do budgeting like she did previously, only now she says things like, "We don't have enough money to pay all the bills" versus the intensity of "We have to get these bills paid! I need more money to do it! How are you going to get the money?" The goal might be the same (pay the bills) but the path to get there is quite different.

Alicia still gets things done, but sometimes they simply take longer to get done. For example, she always writes nice thank you cards for gifts and events which we attend, but she will take a longer time to get them done now than before the stroke. Before, it was like "I need to get this done right now" whereas today it is more like, "Yes, I am going to get that done" but it takes a few days for it to actually happen.

I also find it interesting that Alicia's long-term memory has not been compromised at all. She can remember everything from her life other than losing some of the details, as we all do.

I chose the title of this chapter intentionally to describe the overall result of Alicia suffering a stroke: A healthy but slightly different person.

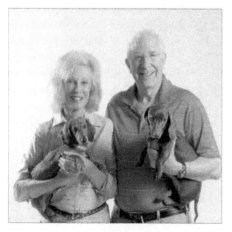

Figure 12-5. Alicia with Bella and the author with Fritzie, our two miniature Dachshunds, taken six months after the stroke in February 2012.

Alicia is as healthy today as she has ever been. But, she is a slightly different person than before: less intense but her skills are the same and her wonderful, natural beauty and magnetic attraction is all there. Here is a wonderful photo of Alicia and me with our two miniature Dachshunds.

Chapter 13

OUR STROKE OF LUCK

"Some guys have all the luck
Some guys have all the pain
Some guys get all the breaks"

Rod Stewart, *Some Guys Have All The Luck*
Reprinted by permission.

The term "Our Stroke of Luck" has many possible meanings. It can mean that you have an inspirational thought, as in hitting your forehead and thinking, "What a stroke of luck to have thought of that." It could mean that you have had a lucky streak betting in Las Vegas as in, "I had a stroke of luck at the Black Jack table last night. I beat the house in ten straight hands." Or, it could mean that you were at the right place at the right time: that the timing of an event was very lucky to have been at one specific time or place.

It is most likely that Alicia had a small bout of atrial fibrillation on either Thursday, August 18, 2011 after returning from a tennis lesson or on Saturday, August 20, 2011 after returning from the Horse

Show in Fairburn, Georgia while napping after being over heated. Temperatures were in the mid-to-upper nineties each day. This is one of the reasons that Atlanta is often referred to as "Hotlanta". If Alicia did have a short bout of atrial fibrillation due to one of these days she was overheated, then it likely caused the formation of a clot that, in turn, caused the stroke.

The clot could have left her heart at any time after it formed. We are extremely lucky that the clot did not dislodge while I was in meetings earlier that day. If so, a number of hours would have passed before I would have returned home to find Alicia either comatose or, worse, deceased. As a result, the timing of the stroke and my coming home from meetings proved to be our stroke of luck. I had talked with Alicia at 6:15 pm. She sounded fine and not likely compromised from a stroke. It appears in retrospect that the entire sequence was truly lucky.

Here are the circumstances that all happened at the right time and in the right sequence on Tuesday, Aug. 23, 2011 and why we believe this was a stroke of luck:

- It was lucky that the clot did not dislodge earlier in the day when I was not at home.
- It was lucky that I got home within fifteen minutes of the onset of the stroke.
- It was lucky that we were able to get Alicia to Northside Hospital within forty-five minutes of the onset of the stroke and within thirty minutes of my finding her.
- It was lucky that we were able to get an initial assessment CAT scan done within an hour of arriving at Northside Hospital that suggested a clot-based stroke.
- It was lucky that Alicia got the tPA treatment started within two hours of the onset of the stroke. The stroke happened around

6:30 pm, and the tPA was started at 8:20 pm, well within the guideline of three hours.

- We were lucky that the attending radiologist was able to find the clot via the MRI within four hours of onset of the stroke.
- We were then lucky to quickly get Alicia transported to the Marcus Stroke Center at Grady Hospital.
- We were lucky that Dr. Raul G. Nogueira had the experience necessary to extract the clot that caused the stroke.
- We were lucky that Dr. Nogueira was able to use the stent retriever device which was then under clinical trial to remove the clot successfully within seven hours of the onset of the stroke.
- We were lucky to have the supervising assistance of Dr. Michael Frankel, Director of the Marcus Stroke Center, and his team to help Alicia in her post-surgical recovery.
- We were lucky to have Dr. Randy Martin, one of the top cardiologists in non-invasive echocardiography, research the cause of the stroke and rule out any underlying, ongoing condition that might require use of life-long blood thinning medication.
- We are lucky to have caring equestrian trainers in Cathy Whiteside, Julie Curtin, Kelly Mullin and John Roper to get Alicia strong enough to ride at the competitive level in the hunter classes over 2' 6" fences in the major horse shows.
- Finally, we were lucky to have the family and friends in our lives who gave Alicia so much support both the night of the onset of the stroke and then following her return home from the hospital.

There are a few other issues that I want to relate about Alicia's recovery from her stroke.

Alicia's (Short-Term) Loss to Her Taste Buds

Alicia suffered an unusual partial loss of her taste buds in November and December 2011. It came on rather suddenly when we were on a vacation in Hawaii. We had scheduled a vacation there to celebrate a wonderful numerical coincidence of November 11, 2011 or "11-11-11." Our lucky numbers have always been 11-11 so we felt that we had to do something special to celebrate 11-11-11.

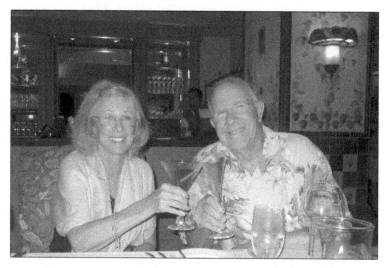

Figure 13.1 Dinner on 11-11-11 at Gaylord's Restaurant, Kilohana Plantation, Kauai. The number sequence represents our lucky numbers so we celebrated it in style.

The loss of taste buds began in Hawaii and continued for about two months. While it came on suddenly one day while we were eating dinner at Roy's in Ko' Olina, Hawaii (on Oahu), it went away rather slowly and did not subside until the end of January.

She told me that a number of things did not taste the way she remembered. Many things simply tasted like cardboard or were bland. While not everything had a different taste, her change in tasted affected most of the things she had always enjoyed. The enjoyment from eating simply went away. Some tastes changed dramatically while others were not affected at all. By Christmas, she reported that some of the old tastes were coming back. By the end of January, she seemed to be back to normal and has not reported that problem again. While we are not one hundred percent sure, we believe the loss of taste buds was related to the stroke recovery.

Alicia's Weight

Alicia has been very weight conscious most of her life. She weighs herself at least twice a day. If she gains two pounds, she cuts back eating, but it is hard to get her to eat more when she loses a pound or two.

Alicia began to lose weight during her recovery from her stroke. While not a lot, but over a number of months, it started to give me some concern, especially if it continued. She lost from a multi-year average of 117 pounds to about 112 pounds.

When her weight began to fall, I began to get concerned. She needed to have enough extra weight over her minimum so she could help fight off infections or a cold or any other malady.

She has made a life commitment to never gain weight. She is absolutely gorgeous and weighs now around what she did in high school. She looks great, but I sense it would be quite detrimental if she lost any additional weight. I admire her for still looking like someone who is half her age.

Back when Alicia went to the University of Georgia, she began to lose weight. Her dad told her if she did not gain ten pounds in the next couple of months, he was taking her out of school. She did not like eating in the university cafeteria so her dad gave her $100 per month to eat out. Slowly, she gained the necessary weight to stay in school.

Alicia told me how happy she was to be shedding a few pounds. When she lost five pounds, I told her she needed to stop losing weight. She has been able to keep herself in the 114-115 range over the years since the stroke.

I think Alicia likes this new, lower weight, but I personally think she is a bit too thin. The point here is that if the person you love starts to lose weight after a stroke, it could be normal, but do not let it go beyond a drop in excess of five percent of the person's body weight, e.g. 5 pounds if 100, 7.5 pounds if 150, etc. Talk to your doctor about it. Do not let it go too far.

One of the issues is that a person needs to have some reserve weight over their minimum to be able to survive surgery or a bad case of the flu. While most people like me need to lose weight, when someone you love loses too much weight, do not let it continue! Make sure that loved one stays above their minimum weight.

Service vs. Independence

The area in which I have had the most difficulty managing regarding Alicia's post stroke recovery is doing things for her as opposed to encouraging her to do them herself. I think that this is a particularly challenging area for me since I was so lucky to get Alicia back into my life forty-five years after we dated in high school. I was lucky to get her back a second time when Dr. Nogueira was able to remove the clot in Alicia's brain that caused her stroke and bring her back to a normal life.

I find that I am constantly doing things for her out of a feeling of service and gratitude. "Here, Honey, let me do that for you." It's a combination of Southern upbringing and appreciation for her being in my life.

We have discussed this issue, it is so ingrained that I often do things automatically rather than think about whether she should do it or not.

Perhaps with her back to being healthy, I can stop doing things for her. Oops, that is not right either! See, it is a difficult issue.

The thing to realize here is that you have to balance loving the post stroke patient, doing things for him or her while recovering from a stroke and encouraging them to do it for themselves. Try to make sure you are challenging that person every day. Yet, do not feel guilty for doing something nice for them. You will feel good seeing them gain confidence and ability to do things. I am sure that I went too far and did too many things for Alicia. However, she is now healthy and I am so grateful.

New Normal

I remember Dr. Frankel telling me at the last checkup that Alicia would make a very good recovery but that she likely would be somewhat different from who she was before the stroke. At first, I did not understand what he meant. My worry was that he was trying to be nice but letting me know that Alicia was not really ever going to be normal again. Actually, he was talking about Alicia coming across as perfectly normal to people that she had never met before. The normal she would be was a slightly different normal than what she was.

I now understand what he meant when he said that. She is certainly normal by any kind of independent evaluation. Anyone who did not know she had a stroke would say that she appears to be "very normal," as determined by the general public.

The best example of this is that she is slightly more mellow or softer in her personality than she used to be. She can now take a small problem on and not make it into a gigantic issue. In the past before the stroke, she would take an issue that was a problem and really focus on it until it was solved. She was relentless about keeping track of money, and if there was a problem, she would focus on it like a hawk and get quite emotional about it until it was solved.

Now, she focuses on many of the same issues but she is a "kinder and gentler" Alicia. I kid her that this has been the one improvement in her personality since the stroke: she is a softer and more relaxed person than before. She still focuses on the problem or issue only now she manages it in a more relaxed manner than before.

Self-Perception

Around six to nine months following the stroke, Alicia began to share that she was able to realize in her consciousness what happened during the stroke. At first, she simply recalled the things that happened on August 23, 2011 when the stroke happened. She began to remember how she felt and what people were saying. For example, she began to recall what she was thinking about when she had the stroke. She remembered trying to get up off the sofa on the porch but could not do it and wondered why she could not do it. And, she remembered coming out of surgery in the ICU.

She has also remembered about the details from just before, during and after her stroke. This was interesting because it gave us an opportunity to consider what most likely caused the clot to form in the first place.

One of the most interesting things happens when Alicia meditates. She reports to me that she can sense an "empty area" inside herself. It's as if the undamaged part of her brain can self-examine and visualize the part of the brain that died as a result of the clot.

The lesson here is to not be shocked if someone you love starts many months later recalling many of the things that happened around the time of the stroke.

Building New Pathways

It is very clear that Alicia has been able to build new pathways through the base of her brain that had become blocked. Some of the pathways could be created and utilized in a matter of minutes while others took a number of months.

As an example, we were taking a tennis lesson and the instructor asked Alicia to serve the ball. She tried to do it as she had done thousands of times before, but the ball went only six to eight inches off her hand. She immediately said, "Whoa – this is strange. I told myself to throw the ball up with my left hand just like I knew how to do before, but it didn't work."

The instructor told her to try really hard to throw the ball very high up with her left hand. It took about ten tries, but eventually Alicia was able to find new pathways to make it work and is now able to serve again like she did before. The same is true for just about any left side function that Alicia knew how to do before. She now has to take a little time to find a new path to make the connection in order to do things as she was able to before the stroke.

The lesson here is that rebuilding new pathways around the damaged area usually can be done to get back to playing a sport or doing a task like taking out contact lens. Sometimes, the new pathway can be found almost immediately, but in many cases it takes a number of months to make it happen. Do not give up. You will likely be able to help the person you love get back to doing most of the tasks he or she was doing before their stroke.

Medical Support System

We are extremely lucky that Alicia suffered her stroke close to the Marcus Stroke Center at Grady Hospital in Atlanta. The following is a photograph of the two most important attending physicians during Alicia's stay at Grady: Dr. Michael Frankel, Director of the Marcus Stroke Center, and Dr. Raul Nogueira, Director, Neuroendovascular Division at the Marcus Stroke and Neuroscience Center who did the actual extraction of the clot in Alicia's lower right brain.

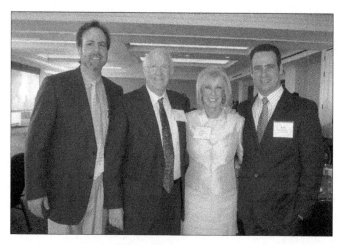

Figure 13-2. Dr. Michael Frankel, Director, Marcus Stroke Center and Professor of Neurology, Emory School of Medicine, Gerry Purdy, AliciaPurdy and Dr. Raul Nogueira, Director, Neuroendovascular Division, Marcus Stroke and Neuroscience Center, Grady Memorial Hospital, Atlanta, Georgia and Professor, Emory School of Medicine, Decatur, Georgia at the Grady Hospital Foundation Luncheon, October 18, 2011.

The Grady team is now doing a lot to promote the stent retriever technique for extracting clots that cause a stroke. Dr. Nogueira has an active Fellowship Program in which he is training other neurosurgeons on the technique extract clots embedded in parts of the brain to more quickly and safely. The Marcus Stroke Center is promoting a number of programs to help stroke centers around the country and the world to have more successful patients like Alicia.

Final Comments

There is one photo sequence that sums up just how lucky we are that Alicia was able to return to full health following her stroke.

The first photo is of Alicia and me taken before the stroke take on June 11, 2008. We were attending our friend Wendy Gifford's sixtieth birthday party at Chez Francois restaurant in Virginia. It was taken by Bob Gifford, Wendy's husband.

The second photo was taken the evening of the day Alicia came home from the hospital on August 27, 2011. Alicia's daughter Sandy and her son Grant were at the house, and the photo was taken by Grant during dinner on the back porch.

The third photo was taken almost two years after the stroke on June 16, 2013 when we were visiting my daughter Jill and her family in Larchmont, NY.

The saying "A picture is worth a thousand words" is very appropriate here. This sequence of three photos clearly shows how Alicia looked before the stroke, what she looked like a few days after the stroke and how she looked about two years after the stroke.

I hope that there can be many more photo sequences like this for those who suffer a stroke. If you are able to manage getting someone who suffers a stroke into a qualified stroke treatment soon after the onset of the stroke, there is a good chance that he or she, too, can fully recover and lead a normal, wonderful life.

You, too, can have your own stroke of luck. You can pay attention to the warning signs and act quickly if you or anyone around you starts to show signs of a stroke.

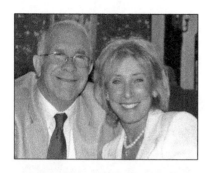

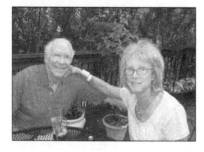

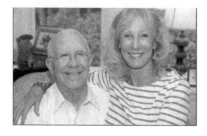

Figure 13-3. This is an absolutely amazing photo sequence. The first photo was taken at our friend, Wendy Gifford's sixtieth birthday party in June 2010. The middle photo was taken in Saturday, August 27, 2011 the afternoon of the day Alicia came home from the hospital. The third photo was taken on June 16, 2013 at my daughter's house in Larchmont, NY during a visit. If you look at the left photo and then the right one, there is no way you could believe that Alicia had suffered a stroke. These three photos represent very graphic proof that it is possible from someone to fully recover from a stroke.

Chapter 14

PERSONAL REFLECTIONS
By Alicia Purdy

The definition of victim is a person who suffers from a destructive or injurious action. That definition makes me a stroke victim. Considering my stroke was serious and injured my entire being, I am not sure what causes one victim to be destroyed and possibly die and another victim to be saved and able to resume a normal life. In my case, I had a severe stroke, but fortunately, I was able to recover and return to the way I lived before the stroke. I am, indeed, very lucky.

My story was owing to "being in the right place at the right time": getting to the Marcus Stroke Center at Grady Hospital in Atlanta in time so that the clot that caused my stroke could be removed in order to give me a chance to recover and return to a normal life.

One thing I can tell you for certain: anyone can have a stroke. It is not like a heart attack that most often comes from the heart's arteries getting clogged up over many years. I kept thinking after the stroke happened to me, "Why in the world did someone like me have a stroke?" You would think I would be the last person that would be afflicted by something like this. I am careful about eating right, about remaining thin, about getting exercise every day, about keeping a low stress profile and about meditating.

What I remember at the time of my stroke was that I was outside sitting on our deck with my cat on one side and my dog on the other. It was very serene, and I remember being thankful for all the colors of the roses and hibiscus and the peacefulness surrounding me. What I did not know was that I was in the process of having a stroke and could not get up to feed the animals. I later learned that there are no nerves that sense pain inside the brain.

As I sat there on the back porch, I did not feel as if anything was wrong! But I noticed that I could not get up. In my mind, I could not figure out why I could not get up. I honestly believed I could get up just like normal so I kept trying to figure out how to do it. I even tried to convince myself that I could get up. I thought, "OK, let's just count 1-2-3 and get up." I tried this but when I said "3" and tried to get up, nothing happened. Later after I recovered I found it interesting that at least part of my brain could still function even though the stroke had already blocked some of the arteries in my brain. Part of my brain was still able to function (thinking) but other parts of my brain (control of my body and muscles) was already compromised.

I realized my husband Gerry was on the way home so I decided to wait so he could lift me up once he arrived. I thought that once he got me up everything would be OK. I still did not think anything was wrong.

I became aware that Gerry had returned home when I heard him calling my name. He came to the back porch and saw where I was sitting. He noticed quickly that something was not right in my responses and asked if I was having any pain. I tried to answer him but realized that I could not verbalize my answer to him because I did not know what was happening to me. All I could do was squeeze out a groan. I felt empty and blank about what to do. However, he immediately knew something was alarmingly wrong and called 911.

I do not have much recollection of being in the Emergence Room at Northside Hospital or being taken to Grady Hospital. I remember I was there and people talking to me, but I find it difficult to remember specific things that were happening. One thing I remember was that when I was at Grady, I kept praying that everything would be OK. I also prayed for my family and friends that that they would all be OK and pray for me.

I do remember waking up in the Intensive Care unit in the Marcus Stroke Center after the procedure to remove the clot. And, I remember Dr. Nogueira showing me on his iPhone the clots that he removed from my brain and Dr. Frankel and Dr. Rivera talking to me about being able to go home just a few days after I was admitted.

When I left the hospital, I remember that I wanted to get back to normal, to be able to remember where I left my keys, my cell phone and the car. It was not always easy to do. One day a few months after the stroke, I went shopping at a Walmart. When I came out of the store, I could not remember where I parked the car so I started pushing the emergency button on the key fob believing it would sound the horn and lights which would show me where the car was located. We all do that coming out of a concert or a sporting event and think nothing of it, that we are smart enough to know how to use the emergency button on the key fob.

But, after the stroke, it was a helpless feeling to walk out and have absolutely no idea where the car was parked. I was not sure if it was on the left, middle or right side. When the emergency button did not sound off, I felt a bit helpless. I called Gerry, and we agreed that would walk from one end of the parking lot to the other pushing the Emergency button every couple of rows. Sure enough, when I got about two thirds of the way through the parking lot, the car's horn sounded and the lights went on and off. I felt relieved but also somewhat angry and disappointed at myself. I realized it was a situation that would not have bothered me before the stroke. That incident caused me to more consciously seek markers near the car when I park the car in a large parking lot.

What was most disturbing me was that I truly did not know where the car was or how to find it. I was very judgmental of myself. When the horn sounded and I saw the car, then the memory of it being where it was came in to my head immediately. I later realized that my brain did not have the connection to tell me where it was, but when I saw the car, my brain made the connection and I knew where it was. I suspect that I was trying to use a part of my brain that had been compromised by the stroke. Normally, that short-term memory of the car's location would be reliable. However, after the stroke, my ability to link to the memory of where the car was located had been compromised. Therefore, I had to find another way to find the car. Walking through the parking lot, pushing the emergency button and then hearing the horn sounding gave me that connection to the memory of where it was located. At that moment, I realized where it was located. It was a strange feeling.

I have tried to use memory techniques to help me build a memory path to find the things I have put down such as my purse, keys and cell phone. Finding the cell phone is easy since you just use another phone to call it. I'll often say, "Gerry, I can't find my phone. Can you please call it?" But, the keys are probably the most difficult since they are small, easy to lose and there is no current easy way to have the key fob issue an audible tone to indicate where they are located. What I have found that helps is either always put them in the same place or try to remember something about where I put them down by verbalizing it in my head. For example, if I put them in the bathroom on the counter, I might say to myself, "OK, I have put the keys in the bathroom. I have to remember they are here and not where I normally put them!"

Also, I have also had a terrible time remembering where I put my glasses. I think all of us who wear glasses often just put them down some place without thinking. Then, a little while later, we want them and cannot remember where we put them. We have had some fun where I tell Gerry, "I can't find my glasses." We then start going through the house and make a game of seeing who can find them first. He wins most of the time and when he finds them, he comes to me with a smile on his face and starts walking me in small baby steps right up to the place where I left them. We laugh and laugh when that happens.

I have a number of friends who have not had a stroke who buy ten to fifteen pairs of glasses and place them all around the house so they just bump into one of them rather than remembering where they are located. Now, I make mental notes that were automatic before the stroke, but I am not complaining because I have become more self-reliant and aware of my surroundings.

The most challenging time for me is when I have put the rose colored glass frames on the rose colored marble counter. Sometimes, I can literally have my hand on the counter just a few inches from the glasses and cannot see them. It is as if they are hidden in the marble. I wonder if the marble hides them from me on purpose!

I wish someone would invent a little, affordable GPS beeper chip that we could put on glasses and keys so we could just call these small devices and have them beep to let us know where they are and, at the same time, show the general location of where they are located on the display of our smartphone. Anyone who can invent this and make it affordable will sell millions of them!

Overall, I am very lucky to have been able to recover from my stroke. I do not think much about it any longer although when I do, it still seems amazing that it happened and just as amazing that I was able to recover.

I am so thankful for the skills of the medical staff at the Marcus Stroke Center at Grady Hospital and to all my friends who have been there with me through my recovery process. I think many of you who read this book will be as thankful as I am to my husband for helping me recover and for writing this book that will be of so much help to others.

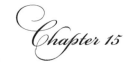

BIBLIOGRAPHY

The following represents both medical journal articles and books on strokes that might be of interest for further learning about strokes and recovery.

Alexander, Eben, MD, <u>Proof of Heaven: A Neurosurgeon's Journey into the Afterlife</u>, Simon & Schuster, 208 pages, ISBN 9781451695182, October 2012. See more at: <u>http://books.simonandschuster.com/Proof-of-Heaven/Eben-Alexander/9781451695182#sthash.gnJ9O0ts.dpuf</u>

Douglas, Kirk, <u>My Stroke of Luck</u>, Harper Collins, Jan 7, 2003, 208p, ISBN 978-0-06-000929-8.

Evans, Robert, <u>The Fat Lady Sang</u>, Harper Collins, Nov. 2013, 184p, ISBN 9781597190305.

Kagan, Jeff, <u>Life After Stroke</u>, <u>On the Road to Recovery</u>, FastPencil, Inc. 2011.

Taylor, Jill Bolte, Ph.D. <u>My Stroke of Insight</u>, <u>A Brain Scientist's Personal Journey</u>, A Plume Book, Penguin Books Ltd, 2009.

The following medical journal articles discuss the type of procedure used to extract the clot in Alicia's brain.

Gupta R, Horev A, Nguyen T, Gandhi D, Wisco D, Glenn BA, Tayal AH, Ludwig B, Terry JB, Hussain MS, Gershon RY, Jovin T, Clemmons PF, Frankel MR, Cronin CA, Tian M, Sheth KN, Anderson AM, Belagaje SR, Nogueira RG. "Higher volume endovascular stroke centers have faster times to treatment, higher reperfusion rates and higher rates of good clinical outcomes." Journal of NeuroInterventional Surgery. 2012 May 13.

Nogueira RG, Smith WS, Sung GY, Duckwiler G, Walker G, Roberts R, Saver J, Liebeskind DS; on Behalf of the MERCI and Multi MERCI Writing Committee. "Effect of Time to Reperfusion on Clinical Outcome of Anterior Circulation Strokes Treated with Thrombectomy: Pooled Analysis of the MERCI and Multi MERCI Trials." Stroke. 2011 Nov; 42(11):3144-9. Epub 2011 Sep 15.

Dipple, et. al. "A Randomized Trial of Intraarterial Treatment for Acute Ischemic Stroke," New England Journal of Medicine, December 17, 2014.

Printed in the USA
CPSIA information can be obtained
at www.ICGtesting.com
JSHW022337140824
68134JS00019B/1539